CONTENTS

Chapter 1: Introduction to Edema — 1
Chapter 2: Anatomy and Physiology of Fluid Balance — 11
Chapter 3: Pathophysiology of Edema — 28
Chapter 4: Types and Etiologies of Edema — 52
Chapter 5: Clinical Manifestations and Diagnosis — 84
Chapter 6: Management and Treatment Approaches — 99
Chapter 7: Complications and Prognosis — 124
Chapter 8: Prevention Strategies and Public Health Implications — 139
Chapter 9: Emerging Research and Future Directions — 159
Chapter 10: Integrative and Holistic Perspectives — 167

CHAPTER 1: INTRODUCTION TO EDEMA

Definition and Overview of Edema

Edema, derived from the Greek word "oídēma" meaning swelling, is a pathological condition characterized by the abnormal accumulation of fluid within the interstitial spaces of tissues, leading to visible swelling or puffiness. It is a common clinical manifestation observed across various medical specialties, ranging from cardiology to nephrology, dermatology to rheumatology.

Understanding Fluid Homeostasis:

To comprehend edema, one must first grasp the delicate balance of fluid dynamics within the human body. The human body comprises several compartments, including intracellular fluid (ICF) within cells and extracellular fluid (ECF) outside cells. The ECF compartment further includes interstitial fluid, plasma, and lymph. Maintenance of fluid balance is crucial for cellular function, tissue integrity, and overall physiological homeostasis.

Pathophysiology of Edema:

Edema arises from disruptions in the intricate mechanisms that regulate fluid movement between these compartments. Several factors contribute to edema formation, including changes in hydrostatic pressure, alterations in oncotic pressure, disturbances in lymphatic drainage, and inflammatory processes. Increased hydrostatic pressure within blood vessels, often seen in conditions like congestive heart failure or venous insufficiency, can lead to fluid leakage into surrounding tissues. Conversely, decreased plasma oncotic pressure, typically due to hypoalbuminemia in conditions such as nephrotic syndrome or liver cirrhosis, promotes fluid extravasation. Lymphatic obstruction or dysfunction impedes the clearance of interstitial fluid, resulting in lymphedema. Additionally, local or systemic inflammation can disrupt endothelial integrity, facilitating fluid leakage and exacerbating edema.

Classification of Edema:

Edema can be classified based on its etiology, anatomical location, duration, and severity. Etiologically, edema can be categorized into various types, including cardiac edema, renal edema, lymphatic edema, and idiopathic edema. Anatomically, it may manifest as peripheral edema (in the limbs), pulmonary edema (in the lungs), cerebral edema (in the brain), or localized edema (in specific organs or tissues). Chronicity distinguishes acute edema, which develops rapidly and resolves within a short timeframe, from chronic edema, which persists over an extended period and may lead to tissue fibrosis and functional impairment. Severity ranges from mild, asymptomatic swelling to severe, debilitating edema associated with complications such as skin breakdown and impaired mobility.

Clinical Presentation and Diagnosis:

The clinical presentation of edema varies depending on its underlying cause, anatomical distribution, and severity. Common signs and symptoms include swelling, pitting or non-pitting edema, weight gain, reduced mobility, and functional impairment. Diagnosis involves a comprehensive medical history, physical examination, and diagnostic studies such as imaging (e.g., ultrasound, MRI) and laboratory tests (e.g., serum albumin, B-type natriuretic peptide). Differential diagnosis is essential to distinguish edema from other conditions presenting with similar symptoms, such as cellulitis, deep vein thrombosis, or lipedema.

Management and Treatment:

Management of edema aims to address the underlying cause, alleviate symptoms, prevent complications, and improve patient outcomes. Treatment strategies may include lifestyle modifications (e.g., dietary sodium restriction, elevation of affected limbs), pharmacological interventions (e.g., diuretics, angiotensin-converting enzyme inhibitors), non-pharmacological therapies (e.g., compression garments, physical therapy), and, in some cases, surgical procedures (e.g., lymphatic surgery, vascular interventions). Multidisciplinary approaches involving physicians, nurses, physical therapists, dietitians, and other healthcare professionals are often necessary to provide comprehensive care and optimize treatment outcomes.

Conclusion:

In summary, edema represents a complex and multifaceted clinical entity characterized by the abnormal accumulation of fluid within tissues. Understanding its pathophysiology, classification, clinical presentation, and management strategies is essential for healthcare providers to effectively diagnose, treat, and manage patients with edema. By addressing the underlying mechanisms and contributing factors, clinicians can mitigate symptoms, improve quality of life, and enhance patient outcomes in individuals affected by this common yet challenging condition.

Classification of Edema: Understanding the Variability in Pathophysiology and Presentation

Edema, a manifestation of fluid imbalance within the body, encompasses a diverse array of etiologies, anatomical distributions, and clinical presentations. A comprehensive classification system is essential to elucidate the underlying mechanisms, guide diagnostic evaluation, and tailor treatment strategies to the specific needs of affected individuals. This exploration delves into the intricate classification of edema, shedding light on its various subtypes and clinical implications.

Etiological Classification:

Edema can be classified based on its underlying cause, which often reflects the primary pathological process driving fluid accumulation. This classification system encompasses several distinct categories, including:

1. **Cardiac Edema:** Resulting from impaired cardiac function, such as congestive heart failure (CHF) or cardiomyopathy, cardiac edema manifests as peripheral swelling, often bilateral and symmetrical in distribution. Elevated venous pressure and diminished cardiac output contribute to fluid retention, leading to systemic congestion and edema formation, particularly in dependent areas such as the lower extremities.
2. **Renal Edema:** Renal disorders, including nephrotic syndrome, acute kidney injury (AKI), and chronic kidney disease (CKD), can disrupt fluid and electrolyte balance, predisposing to edema. Proteinuria,

hypoalbuminemia, and impaired sodium excretion contribute to fluid retention and extracellular volume expansion, culminating in peripheral and periorbital edema.

3. **Hepatic Edema:** Liver dysfunction, as observed in cirrhosis, hepatitis, or hepatic venous congestion, compromises the synthesis of albumin and other plasma proteins essential for maintaining oncotic pressure. Portal hypertension further exacerbates fluid extravasation into the interstitium, resulting in abdominal ascites, lower extremity edema, and pleural effusions.

4. **Lymphatic Edema:** Lymphatic obstruction or dysfunction, whether congenital (e.g., primary lymphedema) or acquired (e.g., lymphadenectomy, radiation therapy), impairs lymphatic drainage, leading to interstitial fluid accumulation. Lymphedema typically presents as unilateral or asymmetric swelling, often affecting the extremities, genitalia, or face, and may be associated with recurrent infections and impaired wound healing.

5. **Idiopathic Edema:** Some individuals may experience recurrent episodes of edema without an identifiable underlying cause, a condition referred to as idiopathic edema. Hormonal fluctuations, dietary factors (e.g., excess salt intake), and venous insufficiency have been implicated in its pathogenesis, although the precise mechanisms remain elusive.

Anatomical Classification:

Edema can also be classified based on its anatomical distribution, providing insights into the underlying pathophysiology and clinical implications. Common anatomical classifications include:

1. **Peripheral Edema:** Predominantly affecting the extremities, peripheral edema manifests as swelling of the hands, feet, ankles, and legs, often accompanied by pitting on palpation. Peripheral edema is commonly associated with conditions such as heart failure, venous insufficiency, and lymphatic obstruction.
2. **Pulmonary Edema:** Involving the accumulation of fluid within the alveoli and interstitial spaces of the lungs, pulmonary edema presents with dyspnea, orthopnea, cough, frothy sputum, and bibasilar crackles on auscultation. Cardiogenic pulmonary edema, typically due to left ventricular failure, and non-cardiogenic pulmonary edema, secondary to acute respiratory distress syndrome (ARDS) or high-altitude exposure, represent distinct etiologies with divergent management strategies.
3. **Cerebral Edema:** Characterized by the abnormal accumulation of fluid within the brain parenchyma or cerebral ventricles, cerebral edema poses significant clinical challenges due to its potential to precipitate intracranial hypertension, herniation, and neurological deterioration. Causes of cerebral edema include traumatic brain injury, ischemic stroke, intracranial hemorrhage, and infectious or inflammatory processes.
4. **Localized Edema:** Occurring in specific organs or tissues, localized edema may arise from localized inflammation, trauma, or obstruction of lymphatic or venous drainage. Examples include macular edema in diabetic retinopathy, periorbital edema in nephrotic syndrome, and scrotal edema in testicular torsion.

Chronicity and Severity Classification:

Chronicity and severity further refine the classification of edema, providing valuable prognostic information and guiding treatment decisions. Acute edema typically develops rapidly and resolves within a short timeframe, often in response to acute insults such as trauma, infection, or surgery. In contrast, chronic edema persists over an extended duration, predisposing to tissue fibrosis, impaired wound healing, and functional impairment. Severity of edema ranges from mild, asymptomatic swelling to severe, debilitating edema associated with complications such as skin breakdown, cellulitis, and venous ulcers.

Conclusion:

In summary, the classification of edema encompasses a spectrum of etiologies, anatomical distributions, chronicity, and severity, reflecting the diverse pathophysiological mechanisms underlying this common clinical entity. A nuanced understanding of these classifications is essential for clinicians to accurately diagnose, stratify risk, and implement tailored treatment strategies aimed at addressing the underlying cause, alleviating symptoms, and optimizing patient outcomes. By elucidating the variability in pathophysiology and presentation, the classification of edema serves as a cornerstone in the comprehensive management of this complex condition.

Epidemiology and Prevalence of Edema: Understanding the Global Burden and Impact

Edema, characterized by abnormal fluid accumulation within tissues, represents a significant public health concern worldwide. Understanding the epidemiology and prevalence of edema is paramount for healthcare professionals, policymakers, and researchers to develop targeted interventions, allocate resources effectively, and mitigate the burden of this pervasive condition. This exploration delves into the epidemiological trends, risk factors, and population characteristics associated with edema, shedding light on its global prevalence and impact on healthcare systems.

Global Burden of Edema:

Edema affects individuals across all age groups, genders, and geographic regions, contributing to morbidity, mortality, and healthcare expenditures. While precise epidemiological data on edema are challenging to ascertain due to variations in definitions, diagnostic criteria, and study methodologies, several population-based studies and systematic reviews provide valuable insights into its prevalence and distribution.

Prevalence Rates and Variability:

The prevalence of edema varies widely across different populations, reflecting differences in underlying risk factors, healthcare infrastructure, and access to care. Studies have reported prevalence rates ranging from 10% to 30% in the general population, with higher rates observed in certain subgroups, such as older adults, individuals with chronic medical conditions, and hospitalized patients. Chronic conditions such as congestive heart failure (CHF), chronic kidney disease (CKD), and venous insufficiency are associated with a higher prevalence of edema due to their impact on fluid homeostasis and cardiovascular function.

Age and Gender Disparities:

Age represents a significant risk factor for the development of edema, with increasing prevalence observed among older adults due to age-related changes in cardiovascular function, renal function, and lymphatic drainage. Gender disparities also exist, with some studies suggesting a higher prevalence of edema in females, possibly attributable to hormonal influences, pregnancy-related changes, and differences in body composition.

Geographic Variations:

Geographic variations in the prevalence of edema reflect differences in socioeconomic status, healthcare infrastructure, and environmental factors. Higher rates of edema have been reported in low- and middle-income countries, where access to healthcare services may be limited, and infectious diseases such as lymphatic filariasis and schistosomiasis contribute to the burden of lymphatic edema. Urbanization, sedentary lifestyles, dietary habits, and environmental pollution further exacerbate the risk of edema in densely populated urban areas.

Risk Factors and Comorbidities:

Several risk factors predispose individuals to the development of edema, including obesity, hypertension, diabetes mellitus, venous thromboembolism, and chronic respiratory diseases. Chronic conditions characterized by fluid retention, such as heart failure, CKD, liver cirrhosis, and nephrotic syndrome, significantly increase the risk of edema due to their impact on renal function, vascular tone, and capillary permeability. Medications such as calcium channel blockers, nonsteroidal anti-inflammatory drugs (NSAIDs), and corticosteroids may also contribute to fluid retention and edema formation.

Clinical and Economic Impact:

Edema imposes a considerable clinical and economic burden on healthcare systems, patients, and caregivers, necessitating comprehensive management strategies to mitigate its adverse effects. Clinically, edema can impair mobility, reduce quality of life, and predispose individuals to complications such as skin breakdown, cellulitis, and venous ulcers. Chronic edema may also lead to tissue fibrosis, lymphedema, and functional impairment, further exacerbating the morbidity associated with this condition. Economically, the direct and indirect costs associated with edema management, including hospitalizations, medications, medical devices, and lost productivity, place a substantial financial strain on individuals, families, and society as a whole.

Conclusion:

In conclusion, edema represents a prevalent and multifaceted clinical entity with significant implications for public health and healthcare delivery. Understanding the epidemiology, prevalence, and risk factors associated with edema is essential for informing preventive strategies, early detection efforts, and targeted interventions aimed at reducing the burden of this condition. By addressing the underlying determinants and modifiable risk factors contributing to edema, healthcare providers can optimize patient outcomes, enhance healthcare system efficiency, and improve population health on a global scale.

CHAPTER 2: ANATOMY AND PHYSIOLOGY OF FLUID BALANCE

Cellular and Tissue Compartments: Exploring the Foundations of Fluid Homeostasis

The human body comprises a complex network of cellular and tissue compartments, each playing a crucial role in maintaining fluid homeostasis, cellular function, and overall physiological equilibrium. Understanding the dynamic interactions between these compartments is essential for comprehending the mechanisms underlying fluid movement, distribution, and regulation within the body. This exploration delves into the intricate anatomy and physiology of cellular and tissue compartments, shedding light on their structural features, functional significance, and contributions to fluid balance.

Intracellular Fluid (ICF) Compartment:

The intracellular fluid (ICF) compartment encompasses the

fluid contained within the cytoplasm of cells, representing the largest reservoir of body water comprising approximately two-thirds of total body water. Within this compartment, water molecules interact with various solutes, including electrolytes (e.g., potassium, magnesium), proteins, carbohydrates, lipids, and metabolic intermediates, facilitating cellular metabolism, enzymatic reactions, and structural integrity. The semi-permeable plasma membrane regulates the movement of water and solutes between the intracellular compartment and the extracellular environment, maintaining osmotic equilibrium and cellular homeostasis.

Extracellular Fluid (ECF) Compartment:

The extracellular fluid (ECF) compartment comprises the fluid outside the cells, including interstitial fluid, plasma, and lymph. Interstitial fluid, the primary component of the ECF, fills the spaces between cells and tissues, providing a milieu for nutrient exchange, waste removal, and cellular communication. Plasma, the liquid component of blood, circulates within the vascular system, transporting oxygen, nutrients, hormones, and metabolic waste products to and from tissues throughout the body. Lymph, derived from interstitial fluid, flows within the lymphatic vessels, serving as a conduit for immune cells, pathogens, and excess fluid to return to the bloodstream.

Endothelial Barrier and Capillary Exchange:

The endothelial barrier, lining the walls of blood vessels and lymphatic vessels, plays a critical role in regulating fluid and solute exchange between the intravascular and extravascular compartments. Endothelial cells form a semi-permeable barrier that selectively permits the passage of water, ions, small molecules, and proteins based on size, charge, and lipid solubility. Capillary exchange, facilitated by processes such as diffusion, filtration, and transcytosis, enables the exchange of nutrients, gases, and metabolic waste products between the bloodstream and surrounding tissues, maintaining tissue perfusion, oxygenation, and nutrient delivery.

Lymphatic System and Fluid Drainage:

The lymphatic system, consisting of lymphatic vessels, lymph nodes, and lymphoid organs, complements the cardiovascular system by regulating fluid balance, immune function, and lipid absorption. Lymphatic vessels collect excess interstitial fluid, protein, and cellular debris from tissues, returning them to the bloodstream via the thoracic duct and right lymphatic duct. Lymph nodes serve as filtration sites, where immune cells monitor for pathogens, toxins, and abnormal cells, initiating an immune response when necessary. Dysfunction of the lymphatic system, as seen in conditions such as lymphedema or lymphatic obstruction, disrupts fluid drainage and predisposes to tissue edema and immune dysfunction.

Renal Mechanisms of Fluid Regulation:

The kidneys play a central role in maintaining fluid and electrolyte balance through processes such as filtration, reabsorption, and secretion. Glomerular filtration within the renal corpuscles generates a plasma ultrafiltrate, which undergoes selective reabsorption of water and solutes along the renal tubules, regulated by hormonal and neurohumoral factors. Antidiuretic hormone (ADH), aldosterone, atrial natriuretic peptide (ANP), and renin-angiotensin-aldosterone system (RAAS) modulate renal tubular function, sodium reabsorption, and water retention, influencing extracellular fluid volume and blood pressure regulation.

Conclusion:

In summary, cellular and tissue compartments constitute the foundation of fluid homeostasis within the human body, orchestrating a delicate balance of fluid distribution, exchange, and regulation to support cellular function, tissue integrity, and physiological equilibrium. The intricate interactions between intracellular and extracellular compartments, facilitated by endothelial barriers, capillary exchange, and lymphatic drainage, ensure dynamic fluid balance and adaptability in response to changing physiological demands. Understanding the anatomy and physiology of cellular and tissue compartments is essential for elucidating the mechanisms underlying fluid imbalance, edema formation, and related pathological conditions, paving the way for targeted interventions and therapeutic strategies aimed at restoring fluid homeostasis and optimizing patient outcomes.

Extracellular Fluid (ECF) and Intracellular Fluid (ICF) Compartments: Key Players in Fluid Homeostasis

Fluid homeostasis, a fundamental aspect of physiological regulation, relies on the dynamic interplay between intracellular fluid (ICF) and extracellular fluid (ECF) compartments. These compartments, each with distinct characteristics and functions, maintain cellular hydration, electrolyte balance, and metabolic integrity essential for overall health and well-being. This exploration delves into the anatomy, composition, regulation, and physiological significance of the ICF and ECF compartments, elucidating their pivotal roles in maintaining fluid balance and cellular homeostasis.

Intracellular Fluid (ICF) Compartment:

The intracellular fluid (ICF) compartment encompasses the fluid enclosed within the cytoplasm of cells, constituting the largest reservoir of body water. Comprising approximately two-thirds of total body water, the ICF plays a central role in cellular metabolism, enzymatic reactions, and structural integrity. Within the ICF, water molecules interact with various solutes, including electrolytes (e.g., potassium, magnesium), proteins, carbohydrates, lipids, and metabolic intermediates, facilitating biochemical processes such as glycolysis, oxidative phosphorylation, and protein synthesis.

Composition and Regulation of the ICF:

The composition of the ICF is carefully regulated to maintain osmotic balance, pH homeostasis, and cellular function. Potassium (K+) is the predominant cation within the ICF, contributing to membrane potential, nerve conduction, and muscle contraction. Magnesium (Mg2+), phosphate (PO4^3-), and organic ions also play essential roles in cellular metabolism and energy production. Intracellular pH is regulated by buffering systems, including proteins, phosphate, and bicarbonate, which maintain the cytoplasmic pH within a narrow physiological range despite fluctuations in metabolic activity and acid-base status.

Extracellular Fluid (ECF) Compartment:

The extracellular fluid (ECF) compartment comprises the fluid outside the cells, encompassing interstitial fluid, plasma, and lymph. Interstitial fluid fills the spaces between cells and tissues, providing a milieu for nutrient exchange, waste removal, and cellular communication. Plasma, the liquid component of blood, circulates within the vascular system, transporting oxygen, nutrients, hormones, and metabolic waste products to and from tissues throughout the body. Lymph, derived from interstitial fluid, flows within the lymphatic vessels, serving as a conduit for immune cells, pathogens, and excess fluid to return to the bloodstream.

Composition and Regulation of the ECF:

The composition of the ECF is finely regulated to maintain osmotic equilibrium, electrolyte balance, and acid-base homeostasis. Sodium (Na+) is the predominant cation in the ECF, exerting osmotic pressure and influencing fluid distribution and blood pressure regulation. Chloride (Cl-) is the primary anion, balancing the charge associated with sodium ions. Bicarbonate (HCO3^-), derived from carbon dioxide (CO2) metabolism, serves as a key buffer system, regulating blood pH and acid-base balance. Hormonal and neurohumoral factors, including aldosterone, antidiuretic hormone (ADH), atrial natriuretic peptide (ANP), and renin-angiotensin-aldosterone system (RAAS), modulate renal tubular function, sodium reabsorption, and water retention, thereby influencing extracellular fluid volume and blood pressure.

Physiological Significance of ICF and ECF:

The ICF and ECF compartments play complementary roles in maintaining cellular hydration, electrolyte balance, and metabolic integrity. Intracellular fluid provides a milieu for cellular metabolism, protein synthesis, and signal transduction, ensuring optimal cellular function and viability. Extracellular fluid facilitates nutrient exchange, waste removal, and communication between cells and tissues, supporting tissue perfusion, oxygenation, and metabolic homeostasis. Dynamic interactions between the ICF and ECF compartments enable adaptive responses to changes in hydration status, osmotic pressure, and metabolic demands, ensuring physiological equilibrium and cellular homeostasis.

Conclusion:

In summary, the intracellular fluid (ICF) and extracellular fluid (ECF) compartments represent essential components of fluid homeostasis, playing integral roles in cellular function, tissue integrity, and physiological equilibrium. Understanding the anatomy, composition, regulation, and physiological significance of these compartments is essential for elucidating the mechanisms underlying fluid balance, electrolyte disorders, and related pathological conditions. By maintaining dynamic interactions between the ICF and ECF compartments, the body ensures optimal cellular hydration, electrolyte balance, and metabolic integrity, thereby promoting health and well-being at the cellular and systemic levels.

The Role of Blood Vessels and Capillary Exchange in Fluid Homeostasis

Blood vessels and capillary exchange play pivotal roles in regulating fluid balance, nutrient delivery, waste removal, and gas exchange throughout the body. The intricate network of blood vessels, comprising arteries, arterioles, capillaries, venules, and veins, facilitates the circulation of blood and the exchange of substances between the bloodstream and surrounding tissues. Capillary exchange, occurring at the level of capillaries, is a dynamic process involving diffusion, filtration, and osmosis, which ensure the exchange of oxygen, nutrients, metabolic waste products, and signaling molecules between the blood and interstitial fluid. This exploration delves into the anatomy, physiology, and regulatory mechanisms governing blood vessels and capillary exchange, elucidating their critical roles in maintaining fluid homeostasis and supporting tissue function.

Anatomy of Blood Vessels:

The cardiovascular system comprises a complex network of blood vessels that deliver oxygen, nutrients, and hormones to tissues and organs throughout the body while removing metabolic waste products and carbon dioxide. Arteries, branching from the heart, carry oxygen-rich blood away from the heart to various tissues and organs. Arterioles, smaller branches of arteries, regulate blood flow and distribute blood to specific tissue beds. Capillaries, the smallest and most numerous blood vessels, form an extensive network of microvessels that facilitate nutrient and gas exchange between the bloodstream and surrounding tissues. Venules and veins collect deoxygenated blood and return it to the heart for reoxygenation and recirculation.

Physiology of Capillary Exchange:

Capillary exchange is the process by which substances are exchanged between the blood and interstitial fluid across the capillary wall. This process occurs through several mechanisms, including diffusion, filtration, and osmosis:

1. **Diffusion:** Small molecules, such as oxygen, carbon dioxide, glucose, and electrolytes, move down their concentration gradients from areas of higher concentration in the blood to areas of lower concentration in the interstitial fluid (and vice versa). This passive process ensures the equilibration of oxygen, nutrients, and metabolic waste products between the bloodstream and surrounding tissues.
2. **Filtration:** Hydrostatic pressure, generated by the pumping action of the heart and the resistance of blood vessels, forces fluid and solutes out of the capillaries into the interstitial space. This process, known as filtration, facilitates the delivery of nutrients, hormones, and oxygen to tissues while removing metabolic waste products and excess fluid from the bloodstream.
3. **Osmosis:** Osmotic pressure, created by the presence of impermeable solutes (such as proteins) in the blood,

draws water into the capillaries from the interstitial space. This osmotic gradient helps maintain plasma oncotic pressure and prevents excessive fluid loss from the bloodstream into the surrounding tissues.

Regulation of Capillary Exchange:

Capillary exchange is tightly regulated by local and systemic factors that modulate vascular tone, blood flow, and permeability. Autoregulation mechanisms, including myogenic response and metabolic regulation, adjust vascular resistance and blood flow in response to changes in tissue oxygenation, metabolic demand, and local factors such as pH, temperature, and mechanical stress. Neurohumoral factors, including sympathetic nervous system activity, circulating hormones (e.g., epinephrine, norepinephrine), and vasoactive peptides (e.g., angiotensin II, endothelin), regulate vascular tone, blood pressure, and capillary permeability, thereby influencing capillary exchange and tissue perfusion.

Clinical Implications of Blood Vessels and Capillary Exchange:

Disorders affecting blood vessels and capillary exchange can have profound clinical implications, ranging from tissue ischemia and hypoxia to edema formation and impaired wound healing. Conditions such as hypertension, atherosclerosis, diabetes mellitus, and peripheral vascular disease can disrupt vascular function, impair capillary exchange, and predispose to tissue damage and organ dysfunction. Edema, characterized by the abnormal accumulation of fluid within tissues, can arise from alterations in capillary permeability, hydrostatic pressure, or osmotic pressure, necessitating comprehensive evaluation and management to address underlying causes and prevent complications.

Conclusion:

In summary, blood vessels and capillary exchange constitute essential components of the cardiovascular system, facilitating nutrient delivery, waste removal, and gas exchange between the bloodstream and surrounding tissues. The intricate anatomy, physiology, and regulatory mechanisms governing blood vessels and capillary exchange ensure optimal tissue perfusion, oxygenation, and metabolic function throughout the body. Understanding the roles of blood vessels and capillary exchange in fluid homeostasis provides insights into the pathophysiology of cardiovascular diseases, vascular disorders, and tissue edema, guiding diagnostic and therapeutic interventions aimed at restoring vascular function and optimizing patient outcomes.

The Lymphatic System: A Vital Component of Fluid Homeostasis

The lymphatic system, often referred to as the body's "second circulatory system," plays a critical role in maintaining fluid balance, immune function, and lipid metabolism. Comprising lymphatic vessels, lymph nodes, lymphoid organs, and lymphatic fluid (lymph), this intricate network serves as a conduit for the transport of interstitial fluid, immune cells, dietary fats, and metabolic waste products. Understanding the anatomy, physiology, and function of the lymphatic system is essential for comprehending its contributions to fluid homeostasis and its implications for health and disease. This exploration delves into the anatomy, physiology, regulation, and clinical significance of the lymphatic system, elucidating its essential role in maintaining fluid balance and supporting immune function.

Anatomy of the Lymphatic System:

The lymphatic system consists of a network of lymphatic vessels that parallel the blood vessels throughout the body. Lymphatic vessels, composed of endothelial cells, collect interstitial fluid, cellular debris, and immune cells from tissues and organs, transporting them to regional lymph nodes for filtration and immune surveillance. Lymph nodes, strategically located along lymphatic vessels, serve as filtration sites where immune cells (e.g., lymphocytes, macrophages) monitor for pathogens, toxins, and abnormal cells, initiating an immune response when necessary. Lymphoid organs, such as the spleen, thymus, tonsils, and adenoids, contribute to immune function by producing, maturing, and activating immune cells in response to antigenic stimuli.

Physiology of the Lymphatic System:

The lymphatic system performs several essential functions that contribute to fluid homeostasis, immune surveillance, and lipid metabolism:

1. **Fluid Balance:** The lymphatic system maintains fluid balance by collecting excess interstitial fluid, protein, and cellular debris from tissues and returning them to the bloodstream via the thoracic duct and right lymphatic duct. This process, known as lymphatic drainage or lymphatic return, helps prevent tissue edema and maintains tissue hydration and integrity.
2. **Immune Function:** Lymphatic vessels and lymph nodes play a crucial role in immune surveillance, defense, and tolerance. Lymph nodes filter lymphatic fluid, removing pathogens, antigens, and abnormal cells, while immune cells within lymphoid organs (e.g., lymphocytes, macrophages) mount an immune response against invading pathogens, toxins, and foreign substances.
3. **Lipid Absorption:** The lymphatic system facilitates

the absorption and transport of dietary fats, fat-soluble vitamins (e.g., A, D, E, K), and cholesterol from the gastrointestinal tract to the bloodstream. Specialized lymphatic vessels called lacteals within the intestinal villi absorb dietary fats and fat-soluble nutrients, forming chylomicrons that are transported via the lymphatic system to the bloodstream.

Regulation of Lymphatic Function:

The lymphatic system is regulated by various mechanisms that modulate lymphatic vessel tone, lymph flow, and immune responses. Smooth muscle cells within lymphatic vessels contract rhythmically, generating lymphatic pulsations that propel lymph forward against gravity. Valves within lymphatic vessels prevent retrograde flow and ensure unidirectional lymphatic drainage. Autonomic innervation, including sympathetic and parasympathetic input, modulates lymphatic vessel tone and lymph flow in response to physiological and pathological stimuli. Hormonal and neurohumoral factors, such as catecholamines, cytokines, and growth factors, regulate lymphatic vessel permeability, immune cell trafficking, and lymphocyte activation, influencing immune responses and tissue inflammation.

Clinical Implications of the Lymphatic System:

Disorders affecting the lymphatic system can have significant clinical implications, including lymphedema, lymphatic obstruction, and impaired immune function. Lymphedema, characterized by the abnormal accumulation of lymphatic fluid within tissues, can result from congenital abnormalities, lymphatic injury (e.g., surgery, trauma), or infectious diseases (e.g., filariasis). Lymphatic obstruction, as seen in conditions such as lymphadenectomy, radiation therapy, or lymphatic malignancies, impairs lymphatic drainage and predisposes to tissue edema, recurrent infections, and impaired wound healing. Immunodeficiency disorders, such as primary immunodeficiencies or acquired immunodeficiency syndrome (AIDS), compromise immune function, impairing the body's ability to mount an effective immune response against pathogens, toxins, and malignant cells.

Conclusion:

In summary, the lymphatic system is a vital component of fluid homeostasis, immune function, and lipid metabolism, playing essential roles in maintaining tissue hydration, immune surveillance, and nutrient transport throughout the body. Understanding the anatomy, physiology, and function of the lymphatic system provides insights into its contributions to health and disease, guiding diagnostic and therapeutic interventions aimed at restoring lymphatic function, optimizing immune responses, and improving patient outcomes. By elucidating the role of the lymphatic system in fluid homeostasis, clinicians can better appreciate its significance in health and disease and develop targeted approaches to manage lymphatic disorders and related conditions.

Renal Mechanisms of Fluid Regulation: Maintaining Fluid and Electrolyte Balance

The kidneys play a central role in regulating fluid and electrolyte balance, ensuring optimal hydration, blood pressure, and metabolic homeostasis within the body. Through processes such as filtration, reabsorption, secretion, and hormonal regulation, the kidneys control the composition and volume of body fluids, excreting waste products and retaining essential substances to maintain physiological equilibrium. This exploration delves into the anatomy, physiology, and regulatory mechanisms governing renal fluid regulation, elucidating the kidneys' essential role in maintaining fluid balance and supporting overall health.

Anatomy of the Kidneys:

The kidneys, paired organs located in the retroperitoneal space, filter blood and regulate fluid and electrolyte balance through the production of urine. Each kidney consists of an outer renal cortex and an inner renal medulla, housing functional units called nephrons. Nephrons comprise a renal corpuscle (glomerulus and Bowman's capsule) and renal tubules (proximal convoluted tubule, loop of Henle, distal convoluted tubule, and collecting duct), where processes such as filtration, reabsorption, and secretion occur. Blood is supplied to the kidneys via the renal arteries, and filtered blood exits via the renal veins.

Physiology of Renal Fluid Regulation:

Renal fluid regulation involves several key processes that influence the composition and volume of urine produced:

1. **Filtration:** Blood enters the kidneys via the renal arteries and is filtered by the glomeruli, specialized capillary networks within the renal corpuscles. Filtration occurs through fenestrated capillary endothelium, basement membrane, and podocyte filtration slits, allowing water, electrolytes, and small solutes to pass into the renal tubules while retaining larger molecules such as proteins and blood cells in the bloodstream.
2. **Reabsorption:** Reabsorption refers to the movement of filtered substances from the renal tubules back into the bloodstream. The proximal convoluted tubule (PCT) is the primary site of reabsorption, where

approximately 65-70% of filtered sodium, water, and other solutes are reabsorbed into the peritubular capillaries. Reabsorption of glucose, amino acids, and bicarbonate also occurs in the PCT, maintaining plasma glucose levels, acid-base balance, and electrolyte concentrations.

3. **Secretion:** Secretion involves the transfer of substances from the peritubular capillaries into the renal tubules for excretion in the urine. Secretion occurs predominantly in the distal convoluted tubule (DCT) and collecting ducts, where hydrogen ions, potassium ions, and organic acids are actively transported into the tubular lumen, contributing to acid-base balance, electrolyte regulation, and toxin elimination.

4. **Hormonal Regulation:** Renal fluid regulation is modulated by hormonal and neurohumoral factors that influence renal tubular function, electrolyte balance, and fluid volume. Key hormones involved in renal fluid regulation include:

Antidiuretic Hormone (ADH): ADH, released from the posterior pituitary gland in response to increased plasma osmolality or decreased blood volume, enhances water reabsorption in the collecting ducts, promoting water retention and urine concentration.

Aldosterone: Aldosterone, secreted by the adrenal cortex in response to decreased blood pressure, sodium depletion, or elevated potassium levels, enhances sodium reabsorption and potassium secretion in the distal tubules and collecting ducts, thereby increasing extracellular fluid volume and blood pressure.

Atrial Natriuretic Peptide (ANP): ANP, released from the atria in response to atrial stretch and increased blood volume, inhibits sodium reabsorption in the distal tubules and collecting ducts, promoting natriuresis, diuresis, and vasodilation, thereby reducing blood volume and blood pressure.

Clinical Implications of Renal Fluid Regulation:

Disorders affecting renal fluid regulation can have profound clinical implications, including volume depletion, electrolyte imbalances, and renal dysfunction. Conditions such as dehydration, hypovolemia, and heart failure can impair renal perfusion and tubular function, leading to decreased urine output, electrolyte disturbances, and fluid overload. Electrolyte imbalances, such as hypernatremia, hyponatremia, hyperkalemia, and hypokalemia, can disrupt cellular function, cardiac conduction, and neuromuscular excitability, potentially resulting in life-threatening complications. Renal diseases, including acute kidney injury (AKI), chronic kidney disease (CKD), and nephrotic syndrome, can compromise renal filtration, reabsorption, and secretion, impairing fluid and electrolyte balance and necessitating comprehensive evaluation and management to prevent further renal damage and optimize patient outcomes.

Conclusion:

In summary, renal mechanisms of fluid regulation play a crucial role in maintaining fluid and electrolyte balance, blood pressure regulation, and metabolic homeostasis within the body. The kidneys, through processes such as filtration, reabsorption, secretion, and hormonal regulation, ensure the optimal composition and volume of body fluids, excreting waste products and retaining essential substances to support cellular function and overall health. Understanding the anatomy, physiology, and regulatory mechanisms of renal fluid regulation provides insights into the pathophysiology of renal disorders, electrolyte imbalances, and fluid disturbances, guiding diagnostic and therapeutic interventions aimed at restoring renal function and optimizing patient outcomes. By elucidating the role of the kidneys in fluid homeostasis, clinicians can better appreciate the significance of renal function in health and disease and develop targeted approaches to manage renal disorders and related conditions.

CHAPTER 3: PATHOPHYSIOLOGY OF EDEMA

Hemodynamic Factors Leading to Edema Formation: Understanding the Fluid Dynamics

Edema, characterized by the abnormal accumulation of fluid within tissues, arises from disruptions in the delicate balance between fluid filtration, distribution, and drainage within the body. Hemodynamic factors, encompassing changes in vascular pressure, permeability, and lymphatic function, play a central role in edema formation by altering fluid dynamics and promoting fluid retention within tissues. This exploration delves into the hemodynamic factors underlying edema formation, elucidating the mechanisms by which alterations in vascular physiology contribute to tissue swelling and fluid imbalance.

Vascular Pressure Dynamics:

Hemodynamic factors influencing edema formation involve alterations in vascular pressures within the microcirculation, including hydrostatic pressure and oncotic pressure:

1. **Hydrostatic Pressure:** Hydrostatic pressure, exerted by the pressure of blood within the blood vessels, drives fluid movement across the capillary membrane. An increase in hydrostatic pressure, as seen in conditions such as venous hypertension or heart failure, promotes fluid filtration from the intravascular space into the interstitial space, leading to tissue edema. Conversely, a decrease in hydrostatic pressure, as observed in hypovolemia or venous insufficiency, impairs fluid reabsorption and predisposes to tissue dehydration and edema resolution.

2. **Oncotic Pressure:** Oncotic pressure, also known as colloid osmotic pressure, is generated by plasma proteins (primarily albumin) within the intravascular space. Oncotic pressure opposes fluid movement out of the blood vessels by exerting an osmotic force that retains water within the intravascular compartment. A decrease in oncotic pressure, secondary to hypoalbuminemia or protein loss, reduces the plasma colloid osmotic gradient, impairing fluid retention and promoting fluid extravasation into the interstitial space, resulting in tissue edema.

Alterations in Vascular Permeability:

Changes in vascular permeability, influenced by inflammatory mediators, endothelial dysfunction, and capillary leak syndrome, contribute to increased capillary permeability and fluid extravasation, predisposing to tissue edema:

1. **Inflammatory Mediators:** Inflammatory mediators, such as histamine, bradykinin, and prostaglandins, induce endothelial cell contraction and intercellular gap formation, leading to increased vascular permeability and protein-rich fluid leakage into the

interstitial space. Inflammatory conditions, including allergic reactions, infection, and autoimmune disorders, can exacerbate capillary leak and promote tissue edema through the release of pro-inflammatory cytokines and vasoactive substances.
2. **Endothelial Dysfunction:** Endothelial dysfunction, characterized by impaired endothelial barrier function and dysregulated vascular tone, disrupts the balance between vasoconstriction and vasodilation, leading to increased capillary permeability and fluid extravasation. Endothelial injury, oxidative stress, and metabolic disturbances contribute to endothelial dysfunction, impairing vascular integrity and promoting tissue edema in conditions such as diabetes mellitus, hypertension, and atherosclerosis.
3. **Capillary Leak Syndrome:** Capillary leak syndrome, characterized by generalized endothelial hyperpermeability and protein-rich fluid extravasation, results in systemic edema and multi-organ dysfunction. Conditions associated with capillary leak syndrome include sepsis, systemic inflammatory response syndrome (SIRS), and cytokine release syndrome (CRS), where excessive cytokine production and endothelial activation lead to widespread vascular leakage and tissue edema.

Lymphatic Dysfunction and Impaired Drainage:

Lymphatic dysfunction and impaired lymphatic drainage contribute to edema formation by disrupting fluid clearance and exacerbating fluid accumulation within tissues:

1. **Lymphedema:** Lymphedema, characterized by impaired lymphatic drainage and protein-rich fluid accumulation within tissues, results from congenital abnormalities, lymphatic obstruction, or secondary

lymphatic dysfunction. Primary lymphedema, such as Milroy disease or lymphatic malformations, arises from developmental defects in lymphatic vessels, while secondary lymphedema can occur secondary to surgery, radiation therapy, infection, or trauma, impairing lymphatic function and promoting tissue edema.
2. **Obstruction:** Lymphatic obstruction, caused by tumors, fibrosis, or lymph node enlargement, impedes lymphatic flow and predisposes to fluid accumulation within tissues. Obstructive lymphedema, such as lymphatic filariasis or lymphadenectomy-related lymphedema, disrupts lymphatic drainage pathways and promotes tissue edema through impaired fluid clearance and protein-rich fluid extravasation.

Clinical Implications and Management Strategies:

Understanding the hemodynamic factors underlying edema formation is essential for the evaluation and management of patients with edematous conditions. Diagnostic modalities, including clinical assessment, imaging studies (e.g., ultrasound, lymphoscintigraphy), and laboratory tests (e.g., serum albumin, inflammatory markers), can aid in identifying underlying etiologies and guiding therapeutic interventions. Management strategies for edema may include addressing underlying conditions (e.g., heart failure, nephrotic syndrome), reducing sodium intake, implementing compression therapy, promoting lymphatic drainage (e.g., manual lymphatic drainage, pneumatic compression devices), and pharmacological interventions (e.g., diuretics, vasopressors, anti-inflammatory agents) to optimize fluid balance and alleviate symptoms.

Conclusion:

In conclusion, hemodynamic factors play a crucial role in edema formation by influencing vascular pressures, permeability, and lymphatic function within the microcirculation. Alterations in hydrostatic pressure, oncotic pressure, vascular permeability, and lymphatic drainage disrupt fluid dynamics and promote fluid accumulation within tissues, leading to tissue edema and clinical manifestations. Understanding the hemodynamic mechanisms underlying edema formation provides insights into the pathophysiology of edematous conditions and guides diagnostic and therapeutic strategies aimed at restoring fluid balance, optimizing vascular function, and improving patient outcomes. By elucidating the complex interplay between hemodynamic factors and edema pathogenesis, clinicians can develop targeted approaches to manage edema and mitigate its impact on patient health and quality of life.

Endothelial Dysfunction and Permeability Changes: Unraveling the Pathophysiology

Endothelial dysfunction, characterized by impaired endothelial barrier function and dysregulated vascular tone, is a hallmark of various pathological conditions affecting the cardiovascular system. Changes in endothelial permeability play a pivotal role in the pathogenesis of edema, inflammation, and tissue injury, contributing to vascular leakage and fluid extravasation into the interstitial space. This exploration delves into the mechanisms underlying endothelial dysfunction and permeability changes, elucidating the complex interplay between endothelial cells, inflammatory mediators, and vascular integrity in health and disease.

Endothelial Structure and Function:

Endothelial cells line the inner surface of blood vessels, forming a dynamic interface between the bloodstream and surrounding tissues. Endothelial cells regulate vascular tone, permeability, and hemostasis by synthesizing vasoactive substances, modulating cell-cell interactions, and responding to mechanical and biochemical stimuli. Endothelial junctions, including tight junctions, adherens junctions, and gap junctions, maintain vascular integrity by regulating paracellular permeability and restricting the passage of solutes and macromolecules across the endothelial barrier.

Mechanisms of Endothelial Dysfunction:

Endothelial dysfunction arises from a myriad of factors that disrupt endothelial barrier function and promote vascular inflammation, including:

1. **Oxidative Stress:** Oxidative stress, resulting from an imbalance between reactive oxygen species (ROS) production and antioxidant defenses, impairs endothelial function by damaging cellular components, including lipids, proteins, and DNA. ROS-mediated endothelial injury leads to increased vascular permeability, leukocyte adhesion, and pro-inflammatory signaling, exacerbating endothelial dysfunction and promoting tissue inflammation.
2. **Inflammation:** Inflammatory mediators, such as cytokines, chemokines, and adhesion molecules, induce endothelial activation and leukocyte recruitment, amplifying vascular inflammation and permeability changes. Inflammatory conditions, including atherosclerosis, sepsis, and autoimmune disorders, trigger endothelial dysfunction by upregulating pro-inflammatory pathways and disrupting endothelial barrier integrity, leading to tissue edema and organ dysfunction.
3. **Shear Stress:** Hemodynamic forces, including shear stress and turbulent flow, exert mechanical strain

on endothelial cells, modulating gene expression, and cellular responses. Prolonged exposure to disturbed flow patterns and oscillatory shear stress promotes endothelial dysfunction by inducing pro-inflammatory signaling, oxidative stress, and endothelial activation, contributing to vascular remodeling and atherosclerotic plaque formation.

Permeability Changes and Vascular Leakage:

Endothelial dysfunction leads to alterations in vascular permeability, characterized by increased paracellular transport and macromolecular leakage across the endothelial barrier:

1. **Tight Junction Disruption:** Endothelial dysfunction disrupts tight junctions, specialized protein complexes that seal intercellular gaps and regulate paracellular permeability. Loss of tight junction integrity permits the passage of solutes, ions, and macromolecules across the endothelial barrier, compromising vascular integrity and promoting fluid extravasation into the interstitial space.
2. **Adherens Junction Dysfunction:** Adherens junctions, composed of vascular endothelial cadherin (VE-cadherin) and associated proteins, maintain cell-cell adhesion and endothelial barrier integrity. Endothelial dysfunction disrupts adherens junctions, leading to increased endothelial permeability and leukocyte transmigration, exacerbating vascular inflammation and tissue injury.
3. **Glycocalyx Degradation:** The glycocalyx, a carbohydrate-rich layer covering the luminal surface of endothelial cells, serves as a molecular sieve and mechanosensor, regulating vascular permeability and endothelial function. Endothelial dysfunction, characterized by glycocalyx degradation and shedding,

compromises vascular integrity and promotes leukocyte adhesion, platelet activation, and thrombus formation, exacerbating tissue inflammation and organ dysfunction.

Clinical Implications and Therapeutic Strategies:

Endothelial dysfunction and permeability changes have significant clinical implications for various cardiovascular and inflammatory disorders, including atherosclerosis, sepsis, acute lung injury, and acute respiratory distress syndrome (ARDS). Therapeutic strategies aimed at preserving endothelial barrier function and mitigating vascular inflammation may include:

1. **Antioxidant Therapy:** Antioxidants, such as vitamin C, vitamin E, and N-acetylcysteine, target oxidative stress and mitigate endothelial dysfunction by scavenging ROS, restoring redox balance, and preserving endothelial integrity.
2. **Anti-inflammatory Agents:** Anti-inflammatory agents, including corticosteroids, nonsteroidal anti-inflammatory drugs (NSAIDs), and biologic agents (e.g., anti-TNF-alpha, anti-IL-6), suppress pro-inflammatory signaling pathways and attenuate endothelial activation, reducing vascular permeability and tissue inflammation.
3. **Endothelial Protective Agents:** Endothelial protective agents, such as statins, angiotensin-converting enzyme (ACE) inhibitors, and endothelial nitric oxide synthase (eNOS) agonists, enhance endothelial function and promote vascular health by modulating nitric oxide (NO) bioavailability, inhibiting endothelial activation, and preserving endothelial barrier integrity.

Conclusion:

In conclusion, endothelial dysfunction and permeability changes play a critical role in the pathogenesis of various cardiovascular and inflammatory disorders, contributing to vascular leakage, tissue edema, and organ dysfunction. Understanding the mechanisms underlying endothelial dysfunction provides insights into the pathophysiology of vascular diseases and informs therapeutic strategies aimed at preserving endothelial barrier function and mitigating vascular inflammation. By elucidating the complex interplay between endothelial cells, inflammatory mediators, and vascular integrity, clinicians can develop targeted approaches to manage endothelial dysfunction and improve patient outcomes in cardiovascular and inflammatory conditions.

Alterations in Osmotic Pressure: Implications for Edema Pathogenesis

Osmotic pressure, a fundamental determinant of fluid distribution and balance within the body, plays a crucial role in regulating fluid movement across cell membranes and vascular compartments. Alterations in osmotic pressure, arising from changes in plasma protein concentration, electrolyte balance, and oncotic gradients, can disrupt fluid homeostasis and contribute to the development of edema. This exploration delves into the mechanisms underlying alterations in osmotic pressure and their implications for edema pathogenesis, elucidating the interplay between osmotic forces, vascular permeability, and fluid distribution in health and disease.

Osmotic Pressure and Fluid Distribution:

Osmotic pressure, governed by the concentration of solutes

within a fluid compartment, exerts an osmotic force that drives water movement across semipermeable membranes. In the context of fluid distribution within the body, osmotic pressure plays a critical role in maintaining fluid balance between intracellular and extracellular compartments, as well as between plasma and interstitial fluid compartments. Plasma proteins, primarily albumin, exert colloid osmotic pressure that opposes hydrostatic forces, retaining water within the intravascular space and preventing excessive fluid extravasation into the interstitial space.

Factors Influencing Osmotic Pressure:

Several factors influence osmotic pressure and contribute to alterations in fluid distribution and edema formation:

1. **Plasma Protein Concentration:** Plasma proteins, particularly albumin, constitute the primary contributors to colloid osmotic pressure within the intravascular space. Decreases in plasma protein concentration, as seen in hypoalbuminemia or protein loss disorders (e.g., nephrotic syndrome, liver disease), reduce colloid osmotic pressure, impairing fluid retention within the intravascular compartment and promoting fluid extravasation into the interstitial space, leading to tissue edema.
2. **Electrolyte Imbalance:** Electrolytes, such as sodium, chloride, potassium, and bicarbonate, influence osmotic pressure and fluid distribution across cell membranes and vascular compartments. Alterations in electrolyte balance, such as hypernatremia, hyponatremia, hyperkalemia, or hypokalemia, disrupt osmotic gradients and fluid equilibrium, predisposing to cellular dehydration or swelling, intravascular volume shifts, and tissue edema.
3. **Oncotic Gradients:** Oncotic gradients, established

by the differential distribution of plasma proteins (primarily albumin) across vascular compartments, regulate fluid movement between the intravascular and interstitial spaces. Disruptions in oncotic gradients, secondary to hypoalbuminemia, protein loss, or capillary leak syndrome, compromise colloid osmotic pressure and fluid retention within the intravascular compartment, facilitating fluid extravasation into the interstitial space and promoting tissue edema.

Edema Pathogenesis:

Alterations in osmotic pressure contribute to edema pathogenesis by disrupting the balance between hydrostatic and oncotic forces within the microcirculation:

1. **Increased Hydrostatic Pressure:** Decreases in colloid osmotic pressure, secondary to hypoalbuminemia or protein loss disorders, reduce the opposing force to hydrostatic pressure, leading to increased capillary filtration and fluid extravasation into the interstitial space. Elevated hydrostatic pressure, as seen in conditions such as venous hypertension or heart failure, further exacerbates fluid retention within tissues, promoting tissue edema and organ dysfunction.
2. **Impaired Oncotic Pressure:** Reductions in colloid osmotic pressure compromise the ability of plasma proteins to retain water within the intravascular space, facilitating fluid leakage across capillary membranes and promoting tissue edema. Impaired oncotic pressure, coupled with increased vascular permeability or lymphatic dysfunction, exacerbates fluid extravasation into the interstitial space, resulting in tissue edema and impaired tissue perfusion.

Clinical Implications and Management Strategies:

Alterations in osmotic pressure have significant clinical implications for various conditions associated with fluid imbalance and edema formation. Management strategies aimed at addressing osmotic disturbances and restoring fluid balance may include:

1. **Albumin Replacement Therapy:** In cases of hypoalbuminemia or protein loss disorders, administration of exogenous albumin may help restore colloid osmotic pressure and improve intravascular fluid retention, thereby reducing tissue edema and improving hemodynamic stability.
2. **Electrolyte Correction:** Correction of electrolyte imbalances, such as sodium, potassium, and bicarbonate abnormalities, is essential for restoring osmotic gradients and fluid equilibrium, thereby mitigating cellular swelling, intravascular volume shifts, and tissue edema.
3. **Diuretic Therapy:** Diuretic agents, such as loop diuretics or thiazide diuretics, may be used to promote renal excretion of excess fluid and electrolytes, thereby reducing intravascular volume overload, decreasing hydrostatic pressure, and alleviating tissue edema.
4. **Nutritional Support:** Adequate nutritional support, including protein supplementation and electrolyte replacement, is essential for addressing osmotic disturbances and supporting fluid balance in patients with hypoalbuminemia or malnutrition-related edema.

Conclusion:

In conclusion, alterations in osmotic pressure play a central role in edema pathogenesis by disrupting fluid distribution, vascular permeability, and tissue hydration within the body. Understanding the mechanisms underlying osmotic disturbances provides insights into the pathophysiology of edematous conditions and informs therapeutic strategies aimed at restoring fluid balance, mitigating tissue edema, and improving patient outcomes. By elucidating the interplay between osmotic forces, vascular integrity, and fluid dynamics, clinicians can develop targeted approaches to manage osmotic disturbances and optimize fluid homeostasis in patients with edema-related disorders.

Lymphatic Obstruction and Impairment: Consequences for Fluid Homeostasis

The lymphatic system, comprising a network of vessels, nodes, and organs, plays a crucial role in maintaining fluid balance, immune function, and lipid absorption within the body. Lymphatic obstruction and impairment, resulting from congenital abnormalities, traumatic injury, or secondary lymphedema, can disrupt lymphatic drainage and promote fluid accumulation within tissues, leading to edema and impaired immune responses. This exploration delves into the mechanisms underlying lymphatic obstruction and impairment, elucidating the consequences for fluid homeostasis, immune function, and tissue health in health and disease.

Anatomy and Physiology of the Lymphatic System:

The lymphatic system functions as a parallel circulatory network that collects interstitial fluid, immune cells, and dietary fats from tissues and organs, transporting them to regional lymph nodes for filtration and immune surveillance.

Lymphatic vessels, composed of endothelial cells, form a network that parallels the blood vessels throughout the body, collecting lymph from tissues and draining it into the lymphatic ducts. Lymph nodes, strategically located along lymphatic vessels, filter lymphatic fluid, removing pathogens, antigens, and cellular debris, while lymphoid organs, such as the spleen and thymus, contribute to immune function by producing and maturing immune cells.

Mechanisms of Lymphatic Obstruction and Impairment:

Lymphatic obstruction and impairment can arise from various causes, including:

1. **Congenital Abnormalities:** Congenital abnormalities of the lymphatic system, such as lymphatic malformations, lymphangiectasia, or primary lymphedema (e.g., Milroy disease), result from developmental defects in lymphatic vessel formation or function. These abnormalities impair lymphatic drainage and predispose individuals to fluid accumulation within tissues, leading to edema and lymphatic dysfunction.
2. **Traumatic Injury:** Traumatic injury, such as surgery, radiation therapy, or trauma, can disrupt lymphatic vessels and impair lymphatic drainage, leading to lymphedema. Surgical procedures involving lymph node dissection or lymphatic vessel disruption, such as lymphadenectomy for cancer treatment, increase the risk of lymphatic obstruction and secondary lymphedema, impairing fluid homeostasis and immune function in affected individuals.
3. **Secondary Lymphedema:** Secondary lymphedema can occur secondary to infections (e.g., filariasis), inflammatory conditions (e.g., cellulitis), or malignancies (e.g., lymphoma, breast cancer).

Infections or inflammation can lead to lymphatic vessel inflammation and fibrosis, impairing lymphatic drainage and promoting fluid accumulation within tissues. Cancer-related lymphedema can result from tumor infiltration or lymph node metastasis, obstructing lymphatic flow and predisposing to tissue edema and lymphatic dysfunction.

Consequences for Fluid Homeostasis:

Lymphatic obstruction and impairment disrupt fluid homeostasis by impairing lymphatic drainage and promoting fluid accumulation within tissues:

1. **Tissue Edema:** Lymphatic obstruction leads to impaired lymphatic drainage and fluid retention within tissues, resulting in tissue edema and swelling. Chronic lymphatic obstruction can lead to fibrosis, adipose tissue deposition, and tissue remodeling, further exacerbating fluid accumulation and impairing tissue function.
2. **Impaired Immune Responses:** The lymphatic system plays a critical role in immune surveillance and defense, with lymph nodes serving as filtration sites where immune cells monitor for pathogens, antigens, and cellular debris. Lymphatic obstruction impairs immune cell trafficking and antigen presentation, compromising immune responses and increasing susceptibility to infections, inflammation, and tissue injury.
3. **Lipid Malabsorption:** The lymphatic system facilitates the absorption and transport of dietary fats and fat-soluble vitamins from the gastrointestinal tract to the bloodstream. Lymphatic obstruction can impair lipid absorption and transport, leading to malabsorption syndromes and nutritional

deficiencies, further compromising overall health and well-being.

Clinical Implications and Management Strategies:

Lymphatic obstruction and impairment have significant clinical implications for various conditions associated with fluid imbalance, immune dysfunction, and tissue injury. Management strategies aimed at addressing lymphatic dysfunction and promoting tissue health may include:

1. **Manual Lymphatic Drainage (MLD):** MLD is a specialized massage technique that promotes lymphatic drainage and reduces tissue edema by stimulating lymphatic vessel contraction and enhancing lymph flow. MLD is commonly used in the management of lymphedema and chronic venous insufficiency to alleviate symptoms and improve tissue health.
2. **Compression Therapy:** Compression therapy involves the application of external pressure to affected limbs or tissues to reduce edema, improve lymphatic circulation, and prevent disease progression. Compression garments, bandages, or pneumatic compression devices can help manage lymphedema and promote tissue healing in individuals with lymphatic obstruction or impairment.
3. **Exercise and Rehabilitation:** Exercise and physical activity promote lymphatic circulation, muscle pump function, and tissue drainage, thereby reducing edema and improving overall lymphatic function. Physical therapy and rehabilitation programs tailored to individual needs can help enhance mobility, reduce swelling, and optimize functional outcomes in patients with lymphatic dysfunction.
4. **Surgical Interventions:** Surgical interventions,

such as lymphaticovenous anastomosis (LVA) or vascularized lymph node transfer (VLNT), may be considered in select cases of lymphatic obstruction or severe lymphedema refractory to conservative management. These procedures aim to bypass obstructed lymphatic pathways or restore lymphatic drainage by transferring healthy lymphatic tissue, thereby improving fluid balance and tissue health in affected individuals.

Conclusion:

In conclusion, lymphatic obstruction and impairment disrupt fluid homeostasis, immune function, and tissue health, predisposing individuals to edema, infections, and impaired wound healing. Understanding the mechanisms underlying lymphatic dysfunction provides insights into the pathophysiology of lymphedema and related conditions, guiding diagnostic and therapeutic strategies aimed at promoting lymphatic drainage, reducing tissue edema, and improving patient outcomes. By elucidating the consequences of lymphatic obstruction on fluid balance, immune responses, and tissue health, clinicians can develop comprehensive management approaches to address lymphatic dysfunction and optimize patient care in affected individuals.

Renal Causes of Edema: Exploring the Nexus between Kidney Function and Fluid Balance

The kidneys play a pivotal role in maintaining fluid and electrolyte balance within the body through intricate processes of filtration, reabsorption, and secretion. Renal dysfunction, arising from various etiologies such as glomerular diseases, tubulointerstitial disorders, or vascular abnormalities, can disrupt these regulatory mechanisms and contribute to the development of edema. This exploration delves into the renal causes of edema, elucidating the pathophysiology, clinical manifestations, and management strategies associated with renal-related fluid imbalance.

Glomerular Diseases:

Glomerular diseases, affecting the filtration function of the kidneys, can lead to proteinuria, hypoalbuminemia, and impaired colloid osmotic pressure, predisposing individuals to fluid retention and edema formation. Conditions such as nephrotic syndrome, characterized by massive proteinuria (>3.5 grams/day), hypoalbuminemia, and generalized edema, disrupt the balance between oncotic and hydrostatic pressures, promoting fluid extravasation into the interstitial space. Mechanisms underlying edema in nephrotic syndrome include reduced plasma oncotic pressure due to protein loss, increased renal sodium retention secondary to activation of the renin-angiotensin-aldosterone system (RAAS), and enhanced capillary permeability due to vascular endothelial dysfunction. Management of nephrotic syndrome-related edema involves sodium restriction, diuretic therapy, and treatment of underlying glomerular pathology to reduce proteinuria and restore renal function.

Tubulointerstitial Disorders:

Tubulointerstitial disorders, affecting the tubular function of the kidneys, can impair fluid and electrolyte regulation, leading to volume overload and edema formation. Conditions such as acute tubular necrosis (ATN), caused by ischemic or nephrotoxic insults, disrupt tubular reabsorption and secretion mechanisms, resulting in impaired fluid excretion and sodium retention. ATN-related edema manifests as oliguric renal failure, volume overload, and peripheral edema, requiring supportive measures such as fluid restriction, diuretic therapy, and management of underlying causes. Chronic tubulointerstitial disorders, such as chronic kidney disease (CKD) or polycystic kidney disease (PKD), can also predispose individuals to fluid imbalance and edema through progressive loss of renal function, electrolyte abnormalities, and impaired urine concentration ability. Management of CKD-related edema involves dietary modifications, blood pressure control, and pharmacological interventions to slow disease progression and alleviate symptoms.

Vascular Abnormalities:

Vascular abnormalities affecting renal blood flow and perfusion can impair renal function and contribute to fluid retention and edema formation. Conditions such as renal artery stenosis, characterized by narrowing of the renal arteries, reduce renal perfusion and activate neurohormonal pathways (e.g., RAAS, sympathetic nervous system), leading to sodium retention, volume expansion, and systemic hypertension. Renal artery stenosis-related edema may manifest as peripheral edema, pulmonary congestion, or resistant hypertension, necessitating revascularization procedures or pharmacological interventions to improve renal blood flow and alleviate symptoms. Other vascular abnormalities, such as renal vein thrombosis or arteriovenous fistulas, can also disrupt renal blood flow and predispose individuals to renal-related edema through impaired venous drainage or arteriovenous shunting, necessitating anticoagulation therapy or surgical interventions to restore vascular patency and renal function.

Systemic Disorders Affecting the Kidneys:

Systemic disorders, such as diabetes mellitus, systemic lupus erythematosus (SLE), or amyloidosis, can affect renal function and contribute to fluid imbalance and edema formation. Diabetes mellitus, characterized by hyperglycemia and microvascular complications, can lead to diabetic nephropathy, characterized by glomerular damage, proteinuria, and renal impairment. Diabetic nephropathy-related edema results from hypoalbuminemia, sodium retention, and vascular endothelial dysfunction, requiring tight glycemic control, blood pressure management, and renoprotective therapies to mitigate renal damage and prevent edema progression. SLE-related nephritis, characterized by immune complex deposition and glomerular inflammation, can lead to lupus nephritis, proteinuria, and renal dysfunction. Edema in lupus nephritis may result from immune-mediated glomerular injury, tubulointerstitial inflammation, or vascular abnormalities, necessitating immunosuppressive therapy, renal biopsy, and multidisciplinary management to preserve renal function and alleviate symptoms.

Conclusion:

In conclusion, renal causes of edema encompass a spectrum of disorders affecting kidney function and fluid balance regulation, including glomerular diseases, tubulointerstitial disorders, vascular abnormalities, and systemic conditions affecting the kidneys. Understanding the pathophysiology, clinical manifestations, and management strategies associated with renal-related fluid imbalance is essential for the evaluation and treatment of edematous conditions. By elucidating the mechanisms underlying renal-related edema, clinicians can develop targeted approaches to address underlying renal pathology, optimize fluid and electrolyte balance, and improve patient outcomes in individuals with renal-related edematous disorders. Early recognition and intervention are crucial for preventing disease progression, reducing complications, and enhancing quality of life in affected individuals.

Inflammatory Pathways in Edema Formation: Unraveling the Immunological Underpinnings

Inflammation, a complex biological response to injury or infection, plays a central role in the pathogenesis of edema by modulating vascular permeability, leukocyte recruitment, and tissue remodeling. Inflammatory pathways orchestrate a cascade of cellular and molecular events that contribute to fluid extravasation, immune cell activation, and tissue edema. This exploration delves into the inflammatory pathways involved in edema formation, elucidating the interplay between inflammatory mediators, endothelial activation, and immune responses in health and disease.

Inflammatory Mediators:

Inflammatory mediators, including cytokines, chemokines, prostaglandins, and histamine, regulate vascular permeability, leukocyte trafficking, and tissue inflammation during the inflammatory response. These mediators are released by activated immune cells, such as macrophages, neutrophils, and mast cells, in response to microbial pathogens, tissue injury, or antigenic stimuli. Cytokines, such as tumor necrosis factor-alpha (TNF-alpha), interleukin-1 (IL-1), and interleukin-6 (IL-6), promote endothelial activation and leukocyte recruitment, exacerbating vascular permeability and tissue edema. Chemokines, such as CCL2 (monocyte chemoattractant protein-1) and CXCL8 (interleukin-8), facilitate leukocyte migration and extravasation into inflamed tissues, amplifying the inflammatory response and promoting fluid accumulation. Prostaglandins, derived from arachidonic acid metabolism, induce vasodilation, vascular permeability, and edema formation through activation of pro-inflammatory signaling pathways. Histamine, released from mast cells and basophils, induces endothelial cell contraction and intercellular gap formation, leading to increased vascular permeability and fluid extravasation into the interstitial space.

Endothelial Activation:

Endothelial cells, lining the inner surface of blood vessels, play a critical role in regulating vascular permeability and fluid homeostasis during inflammation. Endothelial activation, induced by inflammatory mediators and cytokines, leads to the upregulation of adhesion molecules (e.g., E-selectin, P-selectin, ICAM-1) and the release of vasoactive substances (e.g., nitric oxide, prostacyclin). Adhesion molecules facilitate leukocyte-endothelial cell interactions and promote leukocyte adhesion, rolling, and transmigration across the endothelial barrier. Vasoactive substances modulate vascular tone, endothelial permeability, and leukocyte trafficking, contributing to fluid extravasation and tissue edema. Endothelial activation also promotes the production of reactive oxygen species (ROS) and pro-inflammatory cytokines, further exacerbating vascular dysfunction and tissue inflammation.

Leukocyte Recruitment:

Leukocyte recruitment, a hallmark of the inflammatory response, involves a series of adhesive interactions between leukocytes and endothelial cells within the microcirculation. Inflammatory chemokines and adhesion molecules facilitate leukocyte trafficking and extravasation into inflamed tissues, where they contribute to tissue injury, immune surveillance, and host defense mechanisms. Neutrophils, the first responders to inflammation, release proteolytic enzymes, reactive oxygen species, and inflammatory cytokines, promoting tissue damage and edema formation. Macrophages, monocytes, and lymphocytes play a critical role in orchestrating the immune response, phagocytosing pathogens, and producing pro-inflammatory mediators that amplify the inflammatory cascade and exacerbate tissue injury. Dysregulated leukocyte recruitment and activation contribute to the pathogenesis of chronic inflammatory diseases, such as rheumatoid arthritis, inflammatory bowel disease, and atherosclerosis, where persistent inflammation leads to tissue damage, fibrosis, and edema formation.

Tissue Remodeling:

Inflammatory pathways contribute to tissue remodeling and repair processes following injury or inflammation. Fibroblasts, myofibroblasts, and extracellular matrix components play key roles in tissue remodeling, wound healing, and scar formation. Inflammatory cytokines, such as transforming growth factor-beta (TGF-beta), stimulate fibroblast activation and collagen deposition, leading to tissue fibrosis and impaired organ function. Angiogenesis, the formation of new blood vessels, is orchestrated by pro-angiogenic factors, such as vascular endothelial growth factor (VEGF), fibroblast growth factor (FGF), and angiopoietins, in response to tissue ischemia or inflammation. Dysregulated angiogenesis can contribute to tissue edema, neovascularization, and pathological tissue remodeling in chronic inflammatory conditions.

Clinical Implications and Therapeutic Strategies:

Understanding the inflammatory pathways involved in edema formation has important clinical implications for the diagnosis and treatment of inflammatory disorders. Targeted anti-inflammatory therapies, such as corticosteroids, nonsteroidal anti-inflammatory drugs (NSAIDs), and biologic agents (e.g., anti-TNF-alpha, anti-IL-6), can suppress pro-inflammatory signaling pathways and attenuate tissue inflammation, reducing vascular permeability and edema formation. Immunomodulatory agents, such as immunosuppressants, monoclonal antibodies, and cytokine inhibitors, may be used to target specific components of the inflammatory cascade and mitigate tissue injury in autoimmune or inflammatory diseases. Adjunctive therapies, such as anti-oxidants, anti-coagulants, and anti-fibrotic agents, may also be employed to modulate inflammatory responses, restore tissue homeostasis, and promote tissue repair in chronic inflammatory conditions.

Conclusion:

In conclusion, inflammatory pathways play a central role in edema formation by modulating vascular permeability, leukocyte recruitment, and tissue remodeling during the inflammatory response. Understanding the mechanisms underlying inflammation-induced edema provides insights into the pathophysiology of inflammatory disorders and informs therapeutic strategies aimed at targeting specific components of the inflammatory cascade to alleviate tissue inflammation, reduce vascular permeability, and improve patient outcomes. By elucidating the interplay between inflammatory mediators, endothelial activation, and immune responses, clinicians can develop targeted approaches to manage inflammation-related edema and mitigate tissue injury in affected individuals. Early recognition and intervention are crucial for preventing disease progression, reducing complications, and optimizing patient care in inflammatory disorders associated with edema formation.

CHAPTER 4: TYPES AND ETIOLOGIES OF EDEMA

Cardiac Edema: Understanding Congestive Heart Failure and Related Conditions

Cardiac edema, characterized by fluid accumulation in the interstitial spaces of tissues, is a hallmark feature of congestive heart failure (CHF) and related cardiovascular conditions. The intricate interplay between impaired cardiac function, neurohormonal activation, and hemodynamic disturbances contributes to fluid retention, volume overload, and edema formation in individuals with cardiac disease. This exploration delves into the pathophysiology, clinical manifestations, diagnostic evaluation, and management strategies associated with cardiac edema, providing insights into the complex mechanisms underlying fluid imbalance and heart failure syndrome.

Pathophysiology of Congestive Heart Failure:

Congestive heart failure (CHF) is a clinical syndrome characterized by impaired cardiac function, inadequate tissue perfusion, and fluid retention due to structural or functional abnormalities of the heart. Underlying etiologies of CHF include ischemic heart disease, hypertension, valvular heart disease, cardiomyopathies, and myocardial infarction, among others. The pathophysiology of CHF involves a cascade of maladaptive responses, including neurohormonal activation, ventricular remodeling, and impaired myocardial contractility, leading to fluid overload, venous congestion, and tissue edema.

Neurohormonal Activation:

Neurohormonal activation, initiated by reduced cardiac output and arterial underfilling, triggers compensatory mechanisms aimed at restoring tissue perfusion and hemodynamic stability. Activation of the renin-angiotensin-aldosterone system (RAAS) and sympathetic nervous system (SNS) leads to sodium and water retention, vasoconstriction, and increased preload and afterload on the heart. Angiotensin II and aldosterone promote renal sodium reabsorption and potassium excretion, exacerbating volume overload and fluid retention. Sympathetic activation increases heart rate, myocardial contractility, and systemic vascular resistance, further impairing cardiac function and promoting fluid accumulation in tissues.

Ventricular Remodeling:

Ventricular remodeling, characterized by alterations in myocardial structure and function, occurs in response to chronic hemodynamic stress and neurohormonal activation in individuals with CHF. Left ventricular remodeling is characterized by myocardial hypertrophy, fibrosis, and chamber dilation, leading to impaired systolic and diastolic function. Right ventricular remodeling results from increased pulmonary vascular resistance and pressure overload, leading to right ventricular hypertrophy and dysfunction. Ventricular remodeling contributes to progressive heart failure symptoms, including dyspnea, fatigue, and fluid retention, and increases the risk of adverse cardiovascular events, such as arrhythmias and sudden cardiac death.

Impaired Myocardial Contractility:

Impaired myocardial contractility, secondary to ischemia, fibrosis, or cardiomyopathy, reduces cardiac output and systemic perfusion, leading to tissue hypoxia and neurohormonal activation. Contractile dysfunction impairs systolic function, resulting in decreased ejection fraction (EF) and reduced stroke volume, leading to forward failure and inadequate tissue perfusion. Diastolic dysfunction, characterized by impaired ventricular relaxation and compliance, leads to elevated filling pressures and pulmonary congestion, contributing to fluid retention and edema formation. Impaired myocardial contractility is a key determinant of heart failure severity and prognosis, influencing treatment strategies and patient outcomes.

Clinical Manifestations of Cardiac Edema:

Cardiac edema manifests as peripheral and pulmonary symptoms, reflecting fluid accumulation in the interstitial spaces of tissues and organs. Peripheral edema, characterized by swelling of the lower extremities, ankles, or sacrum, results from increased hydrostatic pressure and fluid extravasation into the interstitial space. Pulmonary edema, characterized by dyspnea, orthopnea, and paroxysmal nocturnal dyspnea, results from increased pulmonary capillary pressure and fluid leakage into the alveolar spaces. Other clinical manifestations of cardiac edema include ascites, hepatomegaly, jugular venous distension, and pleural effusions, reflecting systemic congestion and organ dysfunction.

Diagnostic Evaluation:

Diagnostic evaluation of cardiac edema involves a

comprehensive assessment of clinical signs and symptoms, cardiac function, and hemodynamic parameters. Key diagnostic tests include:

1. **Electrocardiography (ECG):** ECG may reveal evidence of cardiac arrhythmias, conduction abnormalities, or ischemic changes suggestive of underlying heart disease.
2. **Echocardiography:** Echocardiography provides detailed assessment of cardiac structure and function, including left ventricular ejection fraction (LVEF), chamber dimensions, valvular function, and diastolic parameters.
3. **Chest X-ray:** Chest X-ray may reveal cardiomegaly, pulmonary congestion, pleural effusions, or interstitial edema suggestive of heart failure.
4. **Biomarkers:** Biomarkers such as brain natriuretic peptide (BNP) and N-terminal pro-BNP (NT-proBNP) are elevated in patients with heart failure and may aid in diagnosis, risk stratification, and monitoring of disease progression.
5. **Hemodynamic Monitoring:** Invasive hemodynamic monitoring with right heart catheterization may be performed in select cases to assess pulmonary artery pressures, cardiac output, and filling pressures, guiding management decisions and therapeutic interventions.

Management Strategies:

Management of cardiac edema involves a multidisciplinary approach aimed at optimizing cardiac function, relieving symptoms, and preventing disease progression. Key management strategies include:

1. **Pharmacological Therapy:** Pharmacological therapy

for heart failure includes diuretics, angiotensin-converting enzyme (ACE) inhibitors, angiotensin receptor blockers (ARBs), beta-blockers, and mineralocorticoid receptor antagonists (MRAs). Diuretics, such as loop diuretics (e.g., furosemide) and thiazides, promote sodium and water excretion, reducing volume overload and relieving symptoms of congestion. ACE inhibitors and ARBs inhibit the RAAS, reducing vasoconstriction, sodium retention, and myocardial remodeling. Beta-blockers improve cardiac function and reduce mortality by antagonizing sympathetic activation and reducing myocardial oxygen demand. MRAs, such as spironolactone and eplerenone, inhibit aldosterone-mediated sodium retention and fibrosis, improving cardiac remodeling and prognosis.

2. **Fluid and Sodium Restriction:** Fluid and sodium restriction are recommended to reduce volume overload and fluid retention in patients with heart failure. Dietary modifications, including limiting salt intake and fluid intake, can help alleviate symptoms of congestion and improve clinical outcomes.
3. **Lifestyle Modifications:** Lifestyle modifications, including weight management, smoking cessation, regular exercise, and alcohol moderation, are recommended to reduce cardiovascular risk factors and improve heart failure outcomes.
4. **Device Therapy:** Device therapy, including implantable cardioverter-defibrillators (ICDs) and cardiac resynchronization therapy (CRT), may be indicated in select patients with heart failure to improve symptoms, reduce hospitalizations, and prolong survival.
5. **Surgical Interventions:** Surgical interventions, such as coronary artery bypass grafting (CABG) or valve

replacement, may be considered in patients with ischemic heart disease or valvular heart disease contributing to heart failure symptoms.

6. **Advanced Therapies:** Advanced therapies, including heart transplantation or mechanical circulatory support (e.g., left ventricular assist devices), may be considered in patients with end-stage heart failure refractory to medical therapy, providing long-term survival and quality of life benefits.

Conclusion:

In conclusion, cardiac edema is a hallmark feature of congestive heart failure and related cardiovascular conditions, reflecting impaired cardiac function, fluid retention, and hemodynamic disturbances. The pathophysiology of cardiac edema involves neurohormonal activation, ventricular remodeling, and impaired myocardial contractility, leading to fluid overload and tissue congestion. Clinical manifestations of cardiac edema include peripheral and pulmonary symptoms, reflecting systemic congestion and organ dysfunction. Diagnostic evaluation involves a comprehensive assessment of clinical signs and symptoms, cardiac function, and hemodynamic parameters. Management of cardiac edema involves a multidisciplinary approach aimed at optimizing cardiac function, relieving symptoms, and preventing disease progression through pharmacological therapy, lifestyle modifications, and device interventions. By elucidating the complex mechanisms underlying cardiac edema, clinicians can develop targeted approaches to manage heart failure syndrome and improve outcomes in affected individuals. Early recognition, timely intervention, and ongoing monitoring are essential for optimizing patient care and reducing morbidity and mortality associated with cardiac edema.

Renal Edema: Exploring Nephrotic Syndrome, Renal Failure, and Renal Impairment

Renal edema, characterized by fluid accumulation in the interstitial spaces of tissues due to impaired renal function, is a hallmark feature of nephrotic syndrome, renal failure, and renal impairment. The kidneys play a crucial role in fluid and electrolyte regulation through processes of filtration, reabsorption, and secretion. Dysfunction of the renal parenchyma, glomeruli, tubules, or interstitium can disrupt these regulatory mechanisms, leading to fluid retention, volume overload, and edema formation. This exploration delves into the pathophysiology, clinical manifestations, diagnostic evaluation, and management strategies associated with renal edema, providing insights into the complex mechanisms underlying fluid imbalance and renal dysfunction.

Pathophysiology of Renal Edema:

Renal edema results from impaired renal function, leading to alterations in fluid and electrolyte balance, hemodynamic disturbances, and neurohormonal activation. Underlying etiologies of renal edema include nephrotic syndrome, acute kidney injury (AKI), chronic kidney disease (CKD), and renal impairment due to structural or functional abnormalities of the kidneys. The pathophysiology of renal edema involves disruption of glomerular filtration, tubular reabsorption, and interstitial fluid dynamics, leading to fluid retention, volume expansion, and tissue congestion.

Nephrotic Syndrome:

Nephrotic syndrome is a clinical syndrome characterized

by massive proteinuria, hypoalbuminemia, edema, and hyperlipidemia, resulting from glomerular injury and increased glomerular permeability. Podocyte dysfunction, immune complex deposition, or genetic abnormalities can lead to glomerular damage, protein leakage, and impaired colloid osmotic pressure, promoting fluid extravasation and tissue edema. Mechanisms underlying edema formation in nephrotic syndrome include reduced plasma oncotic pressure due to protein loss, increased renal sodium retention secondary to activation of the renin-angiotensin-aldosterone system (RAAS), and enhanced capillary permeability due to vascular endothelial dysfunction.

Renal Failure:

Renal failure, encompassing acute kidney injury (AKI) and chronic kidney disease (CKD), results from structural or functional abnormalities of the kidneys, leading to impaired glomerular filtration, tubular reabsorption, and electrolyte regulation. Acute kidney injury is characterized by rapid decline in renal function, resulting from ischemic injury, nephrotoxic insults, or inflammatory conditions. Chronic kidney disease is characterized by progressive loss of renal function over time, resulting from underlying conditions such as diabetes, hypertension, or glomerulonephritis. Impaired renal function in AKI and CKD leads to fluid retention, electrolyte abnormalities, and metabolic disturbances, contributing to volume overload and tissue edema.

Renal Impairment:

Renal impairment due to structural or functional abnormalities of the kidneys can disrupt fluid and electrolyte regulation, leading to volume overload and tissue edema. Conditions such as polycystic kidney disease (PKD), renal artery stenosis, or renal vein thrombosis can impair renal blood flow, glomerular filtration, and tubular function, leading to fluid retention and edema formation. Renal impairment may also result from medication-induced nephrotoxicity, autoimmune disorders, or congenital abnormalities, further exacerbating renal dysfunction and fluid imbalance.

Clinical Manifestations of Renal Edema:

Renal edema manifests as peripheral and pulmonary symptoms, reflecting fluid accumulation in the interstitial spaces of tissues and organs. Peripheral edema, characterized by swelling of the lower extremities, ankles, or sacrum, results from increased hydrostatic pressure and fluid extravasation into the interstitial space. Pulmonary edema, characterized by dyspnea, orthopnea, and paroxysmal nocturnal dyspnea, results from increased pulmonary capillary pressure and fluid leakage into the alveolar spaces. Other clinical manifestations of renal edema include ascites, hepatomegaly, jugular venous distension, and pleural effusions, reflecting systemic congestion and organ dysfunction.

Diagnostic Evaluation:

Diagnostic evaluation of renal edema involves a comprehensive assessment of clinical signs and symptoms, renal function, and hemodynamic parameters. Key diagnostic tests include:

1. **Renal Function Tests:** Renal function tests, including serum creatinine, blood urea nitrogen (BUN), and estimated glomerular filtration rate (eGFR), provide information about kidney function and filtration capacity.
2. **Urinalysis:** Urinalysis may reveal evidence of proteinuria, hematuria, or cellular casts suggestive of underlying renal pathology.
3. **Renal Imaging:** Renal imaging studies, such as ultrasound, computed tomography (CT), or magnetic resonance imaging (MRI), may be performed to assess

renal anatomy, size, and morphology, and identify structural abnormalities or masses.
4. **Renal Biopsy:** Renal biopsy may be indicated in select cases to establish a definitive diagnosis and guide management decisions in patients with suspected glomerular or interstitial disease.

Management Strategies:

Management of renal edema involves a multidisciplinary approach aimed at optimizing renal function, relieving symptoms, and preventing disease progression. Key management strategies include:

1. **Treatment of Underlying Cause:** Treatment of underlying etiologies of renal edema, such as nephrotic syndrome, acute kidney injury (AKI), chronic kidney disease (CKD), or renal impairment, is essential to address the underlying pathology and improve renal function.
2. **Pharmacological Therapy:** Pharmacological therapy for renal edema may include diuretics, angiotensin-converting enzyme (ACE) inhibitors, angiotensin receptor blockers (ARBs), and immunosuppressive agents, depending on the underlying etiology and severity of renal dysfunction.
3. **Fluid and Sodium Restriction:** Fluid and sodium restriction are recommended to reduce volume overload and fluid retention in patients with renal edema. Dietary modifications, including limiting salt intake and fluid intake, can help alleviate symptoms of congestion and improve clinical outcomes.
4. **Renal Replacement Therapy:** Renal replacement therapy, including hemodialysis, peritoneal dialysis, or renal transplantation, may be indicated in patients with end-stage renal disease (ESRD) or refractory

renal failure to maintain fluid and electrolyte balance, remove metabolic waste products, and improve overall survival and quality of life.
5. **Monitoring and Follow-Up:** Close monitoring of renal function, fluid status, electrolyte levels, and hemodynamic parameters is essential to assess response to treatment, detect complications, and optimize management strategies in patients with renal edema.

Conclusion:

In conclusion, renal edema is a hallmark feature of nephrotic syndrome, renal failure, and renal impairment, reflecting impaired renal function, fluid retention, and tissue congestion. The pathophysiology of renal edema involves disruption of glomerular filtration, tubular reabsorption, and interstitial fluid dynamics, leading to fluid accumulation and tissue edema. Clinical manifestations of renal edema include peripheral and pulmonary symptoms, reflecting systemic congestion and organ dysfunction. Diagnostic evaluation involves a comprehensive assessment of clinical signs and symptoms, renal function, and hemodynamic parameters. Management of renal edema involves a multidisciplinary approach aimed at optimizing renal function, relieving symptoms, and preventing disease progression through pharmacological therapy, dietary modifications, and renal replacement therapy. By elucidating the complex mechanisms underlying renal edema, clinicians can develop targeted approaches to manage renal dysfunction and improve outcomes in affected individuals. Early recognition, timely intervention, and ongoing monitoring are essential for optimizing patient care and reducing morbidity and mortality associated with renal edema.

Liver-Related Edema: Unveiling the Intricacies of Cirrhosis and Portal Hypertension

Liver-related edema, characterized by fluid accumulation in the interstitial spaces of tissues, is a hallmark feature of cirrhosis and portal hypertension. The liver plays a pivotal role in fluid and electrolyte homeostasis through processes of detoxification, protein synthesis, and regulation of vascular tone. Dysfunction of the liver parenchyma, hepatocytes, or sinusoidal endothelium can disrupt these regulatory mechanisms, leading to fluid retention, volume overload, and edema formation. This exploration delves into the pathophysiology, clinical manifestations, diagnostic evaluation, and management strategies associated with liver-related edema, providing insights into the complex mechanisms underlying fluid imbalance and hepatic dysfunction.

Pathophysiology of Cirrhosis:

Cirrhosis is a chronic liver disease characterized by progressive fibrosis, nodular regeneration, and distortion of hepatic architecture, leading to impaired liver function and portal hypertension. Underlying etiologies of cirrhosis include chronic viral hepatitis, alcoholic liver disease, non-alcoholic fatty liver disease (NAFLD), autoimmune hepatitis, and genetic disorders. The pathophysiology of cirrhosis involves hepatocyte injury, inflammation, and fibrosis, leading to progressive liver dysfunction and complications such as ascites, hepatic encephalopathy, and variceal bleeding.

Portal Hypertension:

Portal hypertension, a hallmark feature of cirrhosis,

results from increased resistance to portal blood flow and elevated portal venous pressure, leading to splanchnic vasodilation, portosystemic collaterals, and hepatic congestion. The underlying mechanisms of portal hypertension include architectural distortion of the liver, increased intrahepatic vascular resistance, and hyperdynamic circulation. Sinusoidal endothelial dysfunction, hepatic stellate cell activation, and fibrotic deposition contribute to intrahepatic vascular remodeling and increased resistance to portal blood flow, exacerbating portal hypertension and fluid retention.

Hepatic Dysfunction:

Hepatic dysfunction in cirrhosis results from impaired liver function, reduced synthetic capacity, and altered metabolism of toxins and vasoactive substances. Decreased synthesis of albumin and clotting factors leads to hypoalbuminemia and coagulopathy, contributing to fluid extravasation and impaired hemostasis. Altered metabolism of vasoactive substances, such as nitric oxide, endothelin-1, and prostaglandins, disrupts hepatic vascular tone and contributes to splanchnic vasodilation, exacerbating portal hypertension and fluid retention.

Clinical Manifestations of Liver-Related Edema:

Liver-related edema manifests as peripheral and abdominal symptoms, reflecting fluid accumulation in the interstitial spaces of tissues and organs. Peripheral edema, characterized by swelling of the lower extremities, ankles, or sacrum, results from increased hydrostatic pressure and fluid extravasation into the interstitial space. Abdominal distension, ascites, and hepatomegaly result from hepatic congestion and portal hypertension, reflecting systemic congestion and organ dysfunction. Other clinical manifestations of liver-related edema include jaundice, pruritus, encephalopathy, and gastrointestinal bleeding, reflecting liver dysfunction and complications of cirrhosis.

Diagnostic Evaluation:

Diagnostic evaluation of liver-related edema involves a comprehensive assessment of clinical signs and symptoms, liver function tests, imaging studies, and invasive procedures. Key diagnostic tests include:

1. **Liver Function Tests:** Liver function tests, including serum bilirubin, albumin, international normalized ratio (INR), and liver enzymes (AST, ALT, ALP), provide information about liver function, synthetic capacity, and injury.
2. **Imaging Studies:** Imaging studies, such as ultrasound, computed tomography (CT), or magnetic resonance imaging (MRI), may be performed to assess liver morphology, size, and architecture, and identify signs of cirrhosis, portal hypertension, or complications such as ascites or varices.
3. **Doppler Ultrasound:** Doppler ultrasound may be used to assess portal venous flow, hepatic blood flow, and signs of portal hypertension, such as splenic vein dilation or portosystemic collaterals.
4. **Liver Biopsy:** Liver biopsy may be indicated in select cases to establish a definitive diagnosis, assess the severity of fibrosis, and guide management decisions in patients with suspected cirrhosis or liver disease.

Management Strategies:

Management of liver-related edema involves a multidisciplinary approach aimed at optimizing liver function, relieving symptoms, and preventing disease progression. Key management strategies include:

1. **Treatment of Underlying Cause:** Treatment of

underlying etiologies of liver-related edema, such as cirrhosis, chronic viral hepatitis, alcoholic liver disease, or autoimmune hepatitis, is essential to address the underlying pathology and improve liver function.
2. **Diuretic Therapy:** Diuretic therapy, including loop diuretics (e.g., furosemide) and aldosterone antagonists (e.g., spironolactone), is used to promote sodium and water excretion, reduce volume overload, and alleviate symptoms of congestion and ascites.
3. **Paracentesis:** Therapeutic paracentesis may be performed to remove large-volume ascites, relieve symptoms of abdominal distension and discomfort, and improve respiratory function in patients with tense ascites or respiratory compromise.
4. **Albumin Infusion:** Albumin infusion may be used as adjunctive therapy in patients with refractory ascites or spontaneous bacterial peritonitis (SBP) to improve plasma oncotic pressure, reduce renal impairment, and prevent circulatory dysfunction.
5. **Transjugular Intrahepatic Portosystemic Shunt (TIPS):** TIPS may be indicated in select cases of refractory ascites or variceal bleeding to reduce portal hypertension, improve hemodynamic parameters, and alleviate symptoms of portal hypertension and fluid retention.
6. **Liver Transplantation:** Liver transplantation is the definitive treatment for end-stage liver disease and cirrhosis, offering long-term survival and resolution of liver-related complications, including ascites, hepatic encephalopathy, and variceal bleeding.

Conclusion:

In conclusion, liver-related edema is a hallmark feature of

cirrhosis and portal hypertension, reflecting impaired liver function, portal hypertension, and hepatic congestion. The pathophysiology of liver-related edema involves hepatocyte injury, sinusoidal endothelial dysfunction, and hyperdynamic circulation, leading to fluid retention, volume overload, and tissue congestion. Clinical manifestations of liver-related edema include peripheral and abdominal symptoms, reflecting systemic congestion and organ dysfunction. Diagnostic evaluation involves a comprehensive assessment of clinical signs and symptoms, liver function tests, imaging studies, and invasive procedures. Management of liver-related edema involves a multidisciplinary approach aimed at optimizing liver function, relieving symptoms, and preventing disease progression through pharmacological therapy, diuretic therapy, paracentesis, and liver transplantation. By elucidating the complex mechanisms underlying liver-related edema, clinicians can develop targeted approaches to manage hepatic dysfunction and improve outcomes in affected individuals. Early recognition, timely intervention, and ongoing monitoring are essential for optimizing patient care and reducing morbidity and mortality associated with liver-related edema.

Lymphatic Edema: Exploring Lymphedema and Lymphatic Disorders

Lymphatic edema, characterized by fluid accumulation in the interstitial spaces of tissues due to impaired lymphatic function, is a hallmark feature of lymphedema and lymphatic disorders. The lymphatic system plays a crucial role in fluid homeostasis, immune surveillance, and lipid transport through processes of lymph formation, transport, and drainage. Dysfunction of the lymphatic vessels, lymph nodes, or lymphatic capillaries can disrupt these regulatory mechanisms, leading to lymph stasis, protein-rich fluid accumulation, and tissue edema. This exploration delves into the pathophysiology, clinical manifestations, diagnostic evaluation, and management strategies associated with lymphatic edema, providing insights into the complex mechanisms underlying fluid imbalance and lymphatic dysfunction.

Pathophysiology of Lymphatic Dysfunction:

Lymphatic dysfunction can result from congenital abnormalities, acquired conditions, or secondary to surgical interventions, trauma, or infections. Underlying etiologies of lymphatic dysfunction include primary lymphedema (congenital lymphedema), secondary lymphedema (acquired lymphedema), lymphatic malformations, lymphadenectomy, radiation therapy, or inflammatory disorders. The pathophysiology of lymphatic dysfunction involves impaired lymphatic drainage, lymphatic obstruction, or lymphatic leakage, leading to lymph stasis, protein-rich fluid accumulation, and tissue edema.

Primary Lymphedema:

Primary lymphedema, also known as congenital lymphedema, results from developmental abnormalities or genetic mutations affecting the development or function of the lymphatic vessels. Primary lymphedema may present at birth or later in life and is characterized by progressive swelling of the affected limb or body region, lymphedema, and recurrent cellulitis or infections. Genetic mutations affecting genes encoding lymphatic growth factors, receptors, or signaling pathways can disrupt lymphatic development and function, leading to lymphatic dysfunction and tissue edema.

Secondary Lymphedema:

Secondary lymphedema, also known as acquired lymphedema, results from damage or disruption of the lymphatic vessels secondary to surgery, trauma, radiation therapy, infections, or inflammatory conditions. Secondary lymphedema may occur following lymphadenectomy for cancer treatment, trauma to the lymphatic vessels during surgery or radiation therapy, or infection/inflammation leading to lymphatic obstruction or leakage. Secondary lymphedema is characterized by swelling of the affected limb or body region, lymphedema, and predisposition to cellulitis or infections.

Lymphatic Malformations:

Lymphatic malformations are congenital abnormalities of the lymphatic system characterized by dysplastic or aberrant lymphatic vessels, leading to lymphatic obstruction, leakage, or dilation. Lymphatic malformations may present as macrocystic (cystic hygroma), microcystic, or mixed lesions, depending on the size and morphology of the lymphatic channels. Lymphatic malformations can cause lymphatic edema, tissue distortion, or compressive symptoms, depending on the location and extent of the lesion.

Clinical Manifestations of Lymphatic Edema:

Lymphatic edema manifests as swelling, heaviness, and discomfort in the affected limb or body region, reflecting fluid accumulation and tissue congestion. Primary lymphedema typically presents with asymmetric swelling of the affected limb, lymphedema, or body region, with onset in childhood or adolescence. Secondary lymphedema may present with unilateral or bilateral swelling, lymphedema, or tissue edema, following surgery, trauma, or radiation therapy. Lymphatic malformations may present with localized or diffuse swelling, lymphedema, or cystic lesions, depending on the size and location of the lesion.

Diagnostic Evaluation:

Diagnostic evaluation of lymphatic edema involves a comprehensive assessment of clinical signs and symptoms, lymphatic imaging studies, and lymphoscintigraphy. Key diagnostic tests include:

1. **Clinical Evaluation:** Clinical evaluation involves a thorough history and physical examination to assess for signs of lymphatic edema, including swelling, pitting edema, lymphedema, or tissue changes. Assessment of limb circumference, skin texture, and presence of lymphatic channels or collateral vessels may aid in diagnosis.
2. **Lymphatic Imaging:** Lymphatic imaging studies, such as lymphoscintigraphy, magnetic resonance lymphangiography (MRL), or computed tomography (CT) lymphography, may be performed to visualize lymphatic anatomy, identify lymphatic obstruction or leakage, and assess lymphatic function.
3. **Biopsy:** Biopsy of lymphatic tissue or aspirates of cystic lesions may be indicated in select cases to establish a definitive diagnosis, differentiate lymphatic malformations from other vascular lesions, or guide management decisions.

Management Strategies:

Management of lymphatic edema involves a multidisciplinary approach aimed at reducing swelling, alleviating symptoms, and improving lymphatic function. Key management strategies include:

1. **Conservative Therapy:** Conservative therapy for lymphatic edema includes manual lymphatic drainage (MLD), compression therapy, skin care, exercise, and

elevation of the affected limb or body region. MLD involves gentle massage techniques to promote lymphatic drainage and reduce swelling, while compression therapy with compression garments or bandages helps maintain reduced limb volume and prevent recurrent swelling.

2. **Physical Therapy:** Physical therapy modalities, such as exercise, range of motion exercises, and pneumatic compression devices, may be used to improve lymphatic circulation, muscle pump function, and tissue mobility, reducing swelling and improving functional outcomes.

3. **Surgical Interventions:** Surgical interventions for lymphatic edema may include lymphaticovenous anastomosis (LVA), lymph node transfer, or debulking procedures to improve lymphatic drainage, restore lymphatic function, or reduce tissue bulk. LVA involves creating direct connections between lymphatic vessels and adjacent veins to bypass obstructed or damaged lymphatic channels, facilitating lymphatic drainage and reducing swelling.

4. **Sclerotherapy:** Sclerotherapy may be used to treat lymphatic malformations by injecting sclerosing agents into cystic lesions to induce fibrosis and shrinkage, reducing lymphatic leakage and tissue edema.

5. **Medical Therapy:** Medical therapy for lymphatic edema may include diuretics, lymphatic stimulants, or anti-inflammatory agents to reduce swelling, alleviate symptoms, and improve lymphatic function. Diuretics may be used to reduce fluid retention and volume overload in patients with secondary lymphedema or associated conditions such as heart failure or renal dysfunction.

6. **Nutritional Support:** Nutritional support, including

dietary modifications, hydration, and weight management, may be recommended to optimize lymphatic function, reduce inflammation, and promote tissue healing in patients with lymphatic edema.

Conclusion:

In conclusion, lymphatic edema is a hallmark feature of lymphedema and lymphatic disorders, reflecting impaired lymphatic function, fluid stasis, and tissue congestion. The pathophysiology of lymphatic edema involves lymphatic obstruction, leakage, or dysfunction, leading to fluid accumulation and tissue swelling. Clinical manifestations of lymphatic edema include swelling, heaviness, and discomfort in the affected limb or body region, reflecting tissue edema and lymphatic congestion. Diagnostic evaluation involves a comprehensive assessment of clinical signs and symptoms, lymphatic imaging studies, and lymphoscintigraphy. Management of lymphatic edema involves a multidisciplinary approach aimed at reducing swelling, alleviating symptoms, and improving lymphatic function through conservative therapy, physical therapy, surgical interventions, medical therapy, and nutritional support. By elucidating the complex mechanisms underlying lymphatic edema, clinicians can develop targeted approaches to manage lymphatic dysfunction and improve outcomes in affected individuals. Early recognition, timely intervention, and ongoing monitoring are essential for optimizing patient care and reducing morbidity and mortality associated with lymphatic disorders.

Hypoproteinemia-Related Edema: Understanding Protein-

Losing Enteropathy and Malnutrition

Hypoproteinemia-related edema, characterized by fluid accumulation in the interstitial spaces of tissues due to low serum protein levels, is a hallmark feature of protein-losing enteropathy (PLE) and malnutrition. Serum proteins, particularly albumin and globulins, play a crucial role in maintaining oncotic pressure, fluid balance, and tissue integrity. Dysfunction of the gastrointestinal tract, liver, or kidneys can lead to protein loss, reduced protein synthesis, or impaired protein absorption, contributing to hypoproteinemia and fluid retention. This exploration delves into the pathophysiology, clinical manifestations, diagnostic evaluation, and management strategies associated with hypoproteinemia-related edema, providing insights into the complex mechanisms underlying fluid imbalance and protein depletion.

Pathophysiology of Hypoproteinemia:

Hypoproteinemia results from decreased synthesis, increased loss, or altered metabolism of serum proteins, leading to reduced oncotic pressure and fluid extravasation into the interstitial spaces of tissues. Underlying etiologies of hypoproteinemia include protein-losing enteropathy (PLE), liver disease, kidney disease, malnutrition, inflammatory conditions, or genetic disorders. The pathophysiology of hypoproteinemia involves disruption of protein synthesis, absorption, or metabolism, leading to reduced serum protein levels and tissue edema.

Protein-Losing Enteropathy (PLE):

PLE is a condition characterized by excessive loss of serum proteins into the gastrointestinal tract, leading to hypoalbuminemia, hypoproteinemia, and tissue edema. Underlying causes of PLE include inflammatory bowel disease (IBD), celiac disease, lymphatic disorders, intestinal lymphangiectasia, or gastrointestinal malignancies. Dysfunction of the intestinal mucosa, lymphatic vessels, or capillary endothelium can lead to protein leakage, malabsorption, or lymphatic obstruction, contributing to protein loss and fluid retention.

Malnutrition:

Malnutrition is a condition characterized by inadequate intake or absorption of nutrients, including proteins, leading to protein-energy malnutrition (PEM), hypoalbuminemia, and tissue wasting. Underlying causes of malnutrition include inadequate dietary intake, impaired absorption, increased metabolic demands, or chronic illness. Malnutrition can lead to reduced protein synthesis, impaired immune function, and tissue breakdown, contributing to hypoproteinemia and fluid imbalance.

Clinical Manifestations of Hypoproteinemia-Related Edema:

Hypoproteinemia-related edema manifests as peripheral and generalized swelling, reflecting fluid accumulation in the interstitial spaces of tissues due to low serum protein levels. Peripheral edema, characterized by swelling of the lower extremities, ankles, or sacrum, results from decreased oncotic pressure and fluid extravasation into the interstitial space. Generalized edema may involve the face, abdomen, or other body regions, reflecting systemic fluid retention and protein depletion. Other clinical manifestations of hypoproteinemia-related edema include fatigue, weakness, and predisposition to infections, reflecting tissue wasting and immunodeficiency.

Diagnostic Evaluation:

Diagnostic evaluation of hypoproteinemia-related edema involves a comprehensive assessment of clinical signs and symptoms, serum protein levels, nutritional status, and underlying etiologies. Key diagnostic tests include:

1. **Serum Protein Levels:** Serum protein levels, including albumin, total protein, and globulin fractions, provide information about protein status, nutritional status, and potential underlying causes of hypoproteinemia.
2. **Nutritional Assessment:** Nutritional assessment involves evaluating dietary intake, anthropometric measurements, biochemical markers, and functional status to assess nutritional status and identify risk factors for malnutrition or protein depletion.
3. **Endoscopic Evaluation:** Endoscopic evaluation of the gastrointestinal tract may be indicated in patients with suspected PLE to identify mucosal abnormalities, inflammatory lesions, or gastrointestinal malignancies contributing to protein loss.
4. **Imaging Studies:** Imaging studies, such as abdominal ultrasound, computed tomography (CT), or magnetic resonance imaging (MRI), may be performed to assess for structural abnormalities of the liver, kidneys, or gastrointestinal tract suggestive of underlying pathology.
5. **Biopsy:** Biopsy of affected tissues, such as intestinal mucosa, liver parenchyma, or lymph nodes, may be indicated in select cases to establish a definitive diagnosis and guide management decisions in patients with suspected PLE or malnutrition.

Management Strategies:

Management of hypoproteinemia-related edema involves a multidisciplinary approach aimed at addressing underlying causes, replenishing protein stores, and optimizing nutritional status. Key management strategies include:

1. **Treatment of Underlying Cause:** Treatment of underlying etiologies of hypoproteinemia-related edema, such as PLE, liver disease, kidney disease, or malnutrition, is essential to address the underlying pathology and improve serum protein levels.
2. **Dietary Modification:** Dietary modification, including protein supplementation, calorie supplementation, and micronutrient supplementation, may be recommended to improve nutritional status, promote protein synthesis, and prevent further protein depletion.
3. **Enteral Nutrition:** Enteral nutrition via oral supplements, enteral feeding tubes, or parenteral nutrition may be indicated in patients with severe malnutrition or inability to tolerate oral intake, providing essential nutrients, proteins, and calories to support tissue healing and recovery.
4. **Medical Therapy:** Medical therapy for hypoproteinemia-related edema may include albumin infusions, diuretics, anti-inflammatory agents, or immunosuppressive therapy, depending on the underlying etiology and severity of protein depletion.
5. **Nutritional Counseling:** Nutritional counseling and education may be provided to patients and caregivers to promote dietary adherence, optimize nutrient intake, and prevent recurrent malnutrition or protein depletion.
6. **Monitoring and Follow-Up:** Close monitoring of serum protein levels, nutritional status, fluid balance, and clinical symptoms is essential to assess response to treatment, detect complications, and optimize management strategies in patients with hypoproteinemia-related edema.

Conclusion:

In conclusion, hypoproteinemia-related edema is a hallmark feature of protein-losing enteropathy (PLE) and malnutrition, reflecting impaired protein synthesis, absorption, or metabolism, leading to reduced serum protein levels and tissue edema. The pathophysiology of hypoproteinemia-related edema involves disruption of protein homeostasis, fluid balance, and tissue integrity, leading to fluid accumulation in the interstitial spaces of tissues. Clinical manifestations of hypoproteinemia-related edema include peripheral and generalized swelling, fatigue, weakness, and predisposition to infections. Diagnostic evaluation involves a comprehensive assessment of clinical signs and symptoms, serum protein levels, nutritional status, and underlying etiologies. Management of hypoproteinemia-related edema involves a multidisciplinary approach aimed at addressing underlying causes, replenishing protein stores, and optimizing nutritional status through dietary modification, enteral nutrition, medical therapy, and nutritional counseling. By elucidating the complex mechanisms underlying hypoproteinemia-related edema, clinicians can develop targeted approaches to manage protein depletion and improve outcomes in affected individuals. Early recognition, timely intervention, and ongoing monitoring are essential for optimizing patient care and reducing morbidity and mortality associated with hypoproteinemia-related edema.

Medication-Induced Edema: Unraveling Pharmacological Causes and Mechanisms

Medication-induced edema, characterized by fluid accumulation in the interstitial spaces of tissues due to the effects of pharmacological agents, is a common and clinically significant phenomenon encountered in medical practice. A wide range of medications, including cardiovascular drugs, nonsteroidal anti-inflammatory drugs (NSAIDs), corticosteroids, and antidiabetic agents, can contribute to edema formation through various mechanisms. Understanding the pharmacological causes and mechanisms underlying medication-induced edema is essential for clinicians to recognize, prevent, and manage this adverse drug reaction effectively. This exploration delves into the pathophysiology, clinical manifestations, risk factors, and management strategies associated with medication-induced edema, providing insights into the complex interplay between pharmacotherapy and fluid balance.

Pathophysiology of Medication-Induced Edema:

Medication-induced edema can result from a diverse array of pharmacological agents acting on different physiological pathways involved in fluid homeostasis, vascular permeability, and sodium balance. Common mechanisms implicated in medication-induced edema include:

1. **Sodium and Water Retention:** Some medications, such as corticosteroids, nonsteroidal anti-inflammatory drugs (NSAIDs), and certain antihypertensive agents (e.g., calcium channel blockers, vasodilators), can lead to sodium and water retention by altering renal sodium handling, inhibiting prostaglandin synthesis, or modulating vascular tone. Sodium retention increases extracellular fluid volume and hydrostatic pressure, promoting fluid extravasation into the interstitial spaces and edema formation.
2. **Capillary Permeability:** Certain medications, including calcium channel blockers, NSAIDs, and certain chemotherapeutic agents, can increase

capillary permeability by disrupting endothelial cell junctions or promoting the release of vasoactive mediators, such as histamine or bradykinin. Increased capillary permeability facilitates the leakage of plasma proteins and fluid into the interstitial spaces, contributing to tissue edema.
3. **Lymphatic Dysfunction:** Medications that affect lymphatic function or lymphatic drainage, such as tamoxifen, can impair lymphatic vessel contractility, lymphatic flow, or lymphatic clearance, leading to lymphedema and tissue swelling.
4. **Hormonal Imbalance:** Some medications, such as hormone replacement therapy, oral contraceptives, or selective serotonin reuptake inhibitors (SSRIs), can alter hormonal balance and fluid retention, contributing to edema formation.

Clinical Manifestations of Medication-Induced Edema:

Medication-induced edema typically presents as peripheral edema, characterized by swelling of the lower extremities, ankles, or sacrum, reflecting fluid accumulation in the dependent tissues. Other clinical manifestations of medication-induced edema may include:

1. **Generalized Edema:** In some cases, medication-induced edema may manifest as generalized edema involving multiple body regions, including the face, abdomen, or upper extremities, reflecting systemic fluid retention and vascular permeability.
2. **Pulmonary Edema:** Certain medications, such as calcium channel blockers or chemotherapeutic agents, can precipitate pulmonary edema, characterized by dyspnea, orthopnea, and cough, reflecting fluid accumulation in the alveolar spaces and impaired gas exchange.

3. **Ascites:** Medications that promote sodium retention or alter renal function, such as corticosteroids or NSAIDs, may lead to ascites formation in patients with liver disease or congestive heart failure, reflecting fluid accumulation in the peritoneal cavity.
4. **Periorbital Edema:** Some medications, such as calcium channel blockers or corticosteroids, can cause periorbital edema, characterized by swelling around the eyes, reflecting fluid retention and increased vascular permeability in the facial tissues.

Risk Factors for Medication-Induced Edema:

Several factors may increase the risk of developing medication-induced edema, including:

1. **Medication Class:** Certain classes of medications, such as calcium channel blockers, corticosteroids, NSAIDs, and hormone replacement therapy, are commonly associated with edema formation due to their effects on fluid balance, vascular permeability, or lymphatic function.
2. **Dosage and Duration:** Higher doses or prolonged use of medications may increase the risk of developing edema due to cumulative pharmacological effects on fluid homeostasis and tissue permeability.
3. **Underlying Conditions:** Patients with preexisting conditions such as heart failure, liver disease, renal impairment, or lymphatic dysfunction may be more susceptible to medication-induced edema due to underlying alterations in fluid balance, vascular function, or lymphatic drainage.
4. **Concomitant Medications:** Concurrent use of multiple medications with potential edema-inducing effects may synergistically increase the risk of edema formation, particularly in patients with

polypharmacy.

Management Strategies for Medication-Induced Edema:

Management of medication-induced edema involves a multifaceted approach aimed at identifying and mitigating the underlying causes, optimizing pharmacotherapy, and implementing supportive measures to alleviate symptoms and prevent complications. Key management strategies include:

1. **Medication Review:** A thorough review of the patient's medication regimen is essential to identify potential culprits and assess the necessity of each medication. Discontinuation or dose adjustment of offending medications may be considered if clinically appropriate.
2. **Alternative Therapies:** In cases where medication-induced edema cannot be avoided, alternative therapies with lower edema-inducing potential may be considered as substitutes for the offending medication. Switching to alternative pharmacological agents or nonpharmacological interventions may help minimize edema formation while maintaining therapeutic efficacy.
3. **Symptomatic Treatment:** Symptomatic treatment of medication-induced edema may include the use of diuretics to promote fluid excretion, compression therapy to reduce swelling, and elevation of the affected limbs to facilitate venous and lymphatic drainage.
4. **Patient Education:** Patient education plays a crucial role in the management of medication-induced edema, including educating patients about the potential side effects of their medications, signs and symptoms of edema, and strategies for self-management and symptom relief.

5. **Close Monitoring:** Close monitoring of patients receiving medications with potential edema-inducing effects is essential to detect early signs of edema formation, assess treatment response, and adjust management strategies accordingly. Regular follow-up visits and clinical assessments allow for timely intervention and optimization of patient care.

Conclusion:

In conclusion, medication-induced edema is a common and clinically significant adverse drug reaction encountered in medical practice, reflecting the complex interplay between pharmacotherapy and fluid balance. Understanding the pharmacological causes and mechanisms underlying medication-induced edema is essential for clinicians to recognize, prevent, and manage this adverse drug reaction effectively. Medications can contribute to edema formation through various mechanisms, including sodium and water retention, increased capillary permeability, lymphatic dysfunction, and hormonal imbalance. Clinical manifestations of medication-induced edema typically include peripheral edema, generalized edema, pulmonary edema, ascites, and periorbital edema. Several factors, including medication class, dosage, duration, underlying conditions, and concomitant medications, may increase the risk of developing medication-induced edema. Management of medication-induced edema involves a multifaceted approach aimed at identifying and mitigating underlying causes, optimizing pharmacotherapy, and implementing supportive measures to alleviate symptoms and prevent complications. By elucidating the complex mechanisms underlying medication-induced edema, clinicians can develop targeted approaches to recognize, prevent, and manage this adverse drug reaction effectively, optimizing patient care and improving clinical outcomes. Early recognition, timely intervention, and ongoing monitoring are essential for minimizing the impact of medication-induced edema on patient health and well-being.

CHAPTER 5: CLINICAL MANIFESTATIONS AND DIAGNOSIS

Signs and Symptoms of Edema: Understanding the Clinical Manifestations of Fluid Accumulation

Edema, characterized by the abnormal accumulation of fluid in the interstitial spaces of tissues, manifests with a diverse array of signs and symptoms that reflect the underlying pathophysiology, severity, and distribution of fluid accumulation. Recognizing the clinical manifestations of edema is crucial for accurate diagnosis, differential diagnosis, and appropriate management of this common clinical entity. This exploration delves into the signs and symptoms of edema, encompassing peripheral edema, pulmonary edema, cerebral edema, and other systemic manifestations, providing insights into the multifaceted nature of fluid imbalance in clinical practice.

Peripheral Edema:

Peripheral edema, characterized by swelling of the lower extremities, ankles, or sacrum, is one of the hallmark features of edema and is often the most readily observable manifestation in clinical practice. Peripheral edema may present unilaterally or bilaterally and is typically pitting in nature, with indentation of the skin upon palpation. The severity of peripheral edema may vary from mild swelling to marked enlargement of the affected limbs, depending on factors such as the underlying cause, duration, and response to treatment. Common causes of peripheral edema include heart failure, venous insufficiency, renal dysfunction, liver disease, and medications.

Pulmonary Edema:

Pulmonary edema, characterized by fluid accumulation in the alveolar spaces of the lungs, presents with respiratory symptoms such as dyspnea, orthopnea, cough, and frothy pink sputum. Pulmonary edema may result from cardiogenic causes, such as congestive heart failure, myocardial infarction, or valvular heart disease, or non-cardiogenic causes, such as acute respiratory distress syndrome (ARDS), high-altitude pulmonary edema (HAPE), or neurogenic pulmonary edema (NPE). Auscultatory findings in pulmonary edema may include crackles, wheezes, or diminished breath sounds, reflecting underlying lung pathology and impaired gas exchange.

Cerebral Edema:

Cerebral edema, characterized by fluid accumulation within the brain parenchyma or intracranial compartments, presents with neurological symptoms such as headache, altered mental status, seizures, focal neurological deficits, and signs of increased intracranial pressure (ICP). Cerebral edema may result from traumatic brain injury, ischemic stroke, intracerebral hemorrhage, brain tumors, infections, or metabolic disturbances. Clinical assessment of cerebral edema may involve neurological examination, assessment of consciousness level, pupillary response, and signs of meningeal irritation, guiding diagnostic evaluation and management decisions.

Systemic Manifestations:

In addition to peripheral, pulmonary, and cerebral manifestations, edema may present with systemic signs and symptoms that reflect underlying fluid imbalance and organ dysfunction. Systemic manifestations of edema may include:

1. **Weight Gain:** Rapid or excessive weight gain may occur in patients with edema due to fluid retention and volume overload. Monitoring changes in body weight is essential for assessing fluid balance, response to treatment, and disease progression in patients with edema.
2. **Ascites:** Ascites, characterized by fluid accumulation in the peritoneal cavity, presents with abdominal distension, discomfort, and shifting dullness on physical examination. Ascites may result from liver disease, heart failure, renal dysfunction, malignancy, or portal hypertension, necessitating diagnostic evaluation and therapeutic intervention.
3. **Anasarca:** Anasarca refers to generalized edema involving multiple body regions, including the face, abdomen, extremities, and genitalia. Anasarca may occur in severe cases of fluid overload, hypoalbuminemia, or end-stage organ failure, reflecting systemic fluid retention and protein depletion.
4. **Hypertension:** Edema may be associated with hypertension, reflecting volume overload, increased cardiac output, or sodium retention. Monitoring blood pressure is essential for assessing cardiovascular risk, guiding antihypertensive therapy, and optimizing management of edema-associated hypertension.

Differential Diagnosis:

The differential diagnosis of edema encompasses a broad range of medical conditions, including cardiovascular disorders, renal diseases, hepatic dysfunction, venous insufficiency, lymphatic disorders, inflammatory conditions, endocrine disorders, and medication-related adverse effects. A thorough medical history, physical examination, and diagnostic workup are essential for identifying the underlying cause of edema and guiding appropriate management strategies.

Conclusion:

In conclusion, edema presents with a diverse array of signs and symptoms that reflect the underlying pathophysiology, severity, and distribution of fluid accumulation in the body. Peripheral edema, pulmonary edema, cerebral edema, and systemic manifestations are common clinical presentations of edema encountered in medical practice. Recognizing the signs and symptoms of edema is essential for accurate diagnosis, differential diagnosis, and appropriate management of this common clinical entity. A systematic approach to evaluating patients with edema, including comprehensive history-taking, physical examination, and diagnostic evaluation, is essential for identifying the underlying cause, guiding therapeutic interventions, and optimizing patient outcomes. Early recognition, timely intervention, and ongoing monitoring are essential for optimizing patient care and reducing morbidity and mortality associated with edema-related complications.

Diagnostic Modalities for Edema: Utilizing Imaging, Laboratory Tests, and Clinical Evaluation

Accurate diagnosis of edema requires a comprehensive

approach that integrates clinical evaluation, laboratory tests, and imaging modalities to assess the underlying etiology, severity, and extent of fluid accumulation. Various diagnostic tools are available to clinicians to elucidate the cause of edema, differentiate between different types of edema, and guide appropriate management strategies. This exploration delves into the diagnostic modalities for edema, encompassing imaging studies, laboratory tests, and clinical evaluation, providing insights into the multifaceted nature of diagnostic assessment in fluid imbalance disorders.

Clinical Evaluation:

Clinical evaluation forms the cornerstone of the diagnostic workup for edema and involves a comprehensive history-taking, physical examination, and assessment of clinical signs and symptoms. Key components of the clinical evaluation include:

1. **Medical History:** Obtaining a detailed medical history is essential to identify predisposing factors, underlying comorbidities, medication use, recent travel history, occupational exposures, and other relevant information that may contribute to the development of edema. Important historical clues may include the onset, duration, progression, and associated symptoms of edema, as well as exacerbating or alleviating factors.
2. **Physical Examination:** A thorough physical examination is essential to assess the extent, distribution, and characteristics of edema. Key elements of the physical examination include inspection, palpation, percussion, and auscultation of affected body regions to identify signs of fluid accumulation, such as peripheral edema, pulmonary crackles, ascites, or periorbital swelling. Assessment of vital signs, including blood pressure, heart rate,

respiratory rate, and temperature, provides valuable information about hemodynamic status and systemic perfusion.
3. **Assessment of Fluid Balance:** Evaluation of fluid balance involves assessing intake and output, including oral intake, urine output, insensible losses, and fluid retention. Monitoring changes in body weight, peripheral edema, and ascites can provide valuable insights into fluid status and response to treatment.

Laboratory Tests:

Laboratory tests play a crucial role in the diagnostic evaluation of edema and may include routine blood tests, serum biomarkers, urine studies, and specialized tests tailored to the underlying etiology. Common laboratory tests used in the assessment of edema include:

1. **Complete Blood Count (CBC):** CBC with differential provides information about hematological parameters, including hemoglobin, hematocrit, white blood cell count, and platelet count, which may be useful in identifying underlying causes of edema, such as anemia, infection, or inflammatory conditions.
2. **Electrolyte Panel:** Electrolyte panel assesses serum levels of sodium, potassium, chloride, bicarbonate, calcium, and magnesium, providing insights into electrolyte balance, renal function, and acid-base status, which may be perturbed in patients with fluid imbalance.
3. **Renal Function Tests:** Renal function tests, including serum creatinine, blood urea nitrogen (BUN), and estimated glomerular filtration rate (eGFR), assess renal function and filtration capacity, which are important determinants of fluid balance and

electrolyte homeostasis.
4. **Liver Function Tests:** Liver function tests, including serum levels of transaminases (AST, ALT), alkaline phosphatase (ALP), bilirubin, and albumin, evaluate hepatic function and synthetic capacity, which may be impaired in patients with liver disease or congestive hepatopathy contributing to edema.
5. **Serum Protein Levels:** Measurement of serum protein levels, including total protein, albumin, and globulin fractions, provides information about protein status, nutritional status, and potential causes of hypoproteinemia-related edema.
6. **Inflammatory Markers:** Measurement of inflammatory markers, such as C-reactive protein (CRP) and erythrocyte sedimentation rate (ESR), may be useful in assessing the degree of inflammation and underlying inflammatory conditions associated with edema.
7. **Urinalysis:** Urinalysis evaluates urine characteristics, including color, clarity, specific gravity, pH, protein, glucose, ketones, blood, and sediment, which may provide clues to renal function, urinary tract abnormalities, or proteinuria associated with edema.

Imaging Studies:

Imaging studies play a pivotal role in the diagnostic assessment of edema and may include a variety of modalities, such as:

1. **X-ray:** Plain radiography, including chest X-ray and extremity X-ray, may be performed to assess for pulmonary congestion, pleural effusions, cardiomegaly, bone abnormalities, or soft tissue swelling associated with edema.
2. **Ultrasound:** Ultrasonography is a non-invasive imaging modality that can assess fluid accumulation,

organ size, vascular patency, and structural abnormalities. Ultrasonography may be used to evaluate peripheral edema, ascites, pleural effusions, hepatomegaly, or renal abnormalities contributing to edema.

3. **Computed Tomography (CT):** CT imaging provides detailed anatomical information and may be used to assess for visceral edema, lymphadenopathy, tumor masses, abscesses, or other structural abnormalities associated with edema.
4. **Magnetic Resonance Imaging (MRI):** MRI offers superior soft tissue contrast and may be indicated for evaluating cerebral edema, spinal cord compression, or soft tissue abnormalities not well visualized on other imaging modalities.
5. **Echocardiography:** Echocardiography is a valuable tool for assessing cardiac structure and function, including left ventricular ejection fraction, valvular abnormalities, pericardial effusion, and signs of congestive heart failure contributing to edema.
6. **Lymphoscintigraphy:** Lymphoscintigraphy is a specialized imaging technique used to evaluate lymphatic function, lymphatic drainage patterns, and lymphatic obstruction in patients with lymphedema or suspected lymphatic disorders.

Specialized Tests:

In addition to routine laboratory tests and imaging studies, specialized tests may be indicated based on the suspected underlying etiology of edema. These may include:

1. **Cardiac Biomarkers:** Measurement of cardiac biomarkers, such as brain natriuretic peptide (BNP) or N-terminal pro-BNP (NT-proBNP), may be useful in assessing cardiac function, identifying heart failure,

or evaluating pulmonary edema.
2. **Pulmonary Function Tests:** Pulmonary function tests, including spirometry, lung volumes, and diffusion capacity, may be performed to assess respiratory function, identify pulmonary edema, or evaluate underlying lung disease.
3. **Endoscopic Evaluation:** Endoscopic evaluation of the gastrointestinal tract may be indicated in patients with suspected protein-losing enteropathy (PLE) to identify mucosal abnormalities, inflammatory lesions, or gastrointestinal malignancies contributing to protein loss and edema.
4. **Biopsy:** Biopsy of affected tissues, such as skin, liver, kidney, or lymph nodes, may be indicated in select cases to establish a definitive diagnosis, differentiate between different types of edema, or guide management decisions.

Conclusion:

In conclusion, the diagnostic evaluation of edema encompasses a comprehensive approach that integrates clinical evaluation, laboratory tests, imaging studies, and specialized tests to assess the underlying etiology, severity, and extent of fluid accumulation. Clinical evaluation involves a detailed medical history, physical examination, and assessment of clinical signs and symptoms. Laboratory tests provide valuable information about hematological parameters, electrolyte balance, renal function, hepatic function, serum protein levels, and inflammatory markers. Imaging studies offer detailed anatomical information and may include X-ray, ultrasound, CT, MRI, echocardiography, and lymphoscintigraphy. Specialized tests may be indicated based on the suspected underlying etiology of edema, such as cardiac biomarkers, pulmonary function tests, endoscopic evaluation, or biopsy. A systematic approach to diagnostic assessment is essential for accurate diagnosis, differential diagnosis, and appropriate management of edema, optimizing patient care and improving clinical outcomes. Early recognition, timely intervention, and ongoing monitoring are essential for optimizing patient care and reducing morbidity and mortality associated with edema-related complications.

Exploring the Differential Diagnosis of Edema: Unraveling Underlying Etiologies

Edema, characterized by abnormal accumulation of fluid in the interstitial spaces of tissues, presents with a myriad of clinical manifestations that can result from diverse underlying etiologies. Differential diagnosis of edema involves a systematic approach to identify the primary cause, contributing factors, and associated conditions that may precipitate fluid imbalance. This exploration delves into the differential diagnosis of edema, encompassing cardiovascular disorders, renal diseases, hepatic dysfunction, venous insufficiency, lymphatic disorders, inflammatory conditions, endocrine disorders, medication-related adverse effects, and other less common etiologies, providing insights into the multifaceted nature of fluid imbalance disorders in clinical practice.

Cardiovascular Disorders:

Cardiovascular disorders represent one of the most common etiologies of edema and may include:

1. **Congestive Heart Failure (CHF):** CHF is characterized by impaired cardiac function leading to fluid retention, pulmonary congestion, and peripheral edema. Clinical features of CHF-related edema may include bilateral lower extremity edema, orthopnea,

paroxysmal nocturnal dyspnea, and signs of volume overload on physical examination.
2. **Cardiomyopathy:** Cardiomyopathy, including dilated cardiomyopathy, hypertrophic cardiomyopathy, or restrictive cardiomyopathy, may lead to impaired myocardial function, reduced cardiac output, and fluid accumulation. Edema may be present in patients with advanced cardiomyopathy and signs of heart failure.
3. **Valvular Heart Disease:** Valvular heart disease, such as mitral valve regurgitation, aortic valve stenosis, or tricuspid valve insufficiency, can result in volume overload, pulmonary congestion, and peripheral edema. Examination findings may include jugular venous distention, pulmonary crackles, and dependent edema.

Renal Diseases:

Renal diseases are a common cause of edema and may include:

1. **Acute Kidney Injury (AKI):** AKI, characterized by sudden loss of renal function, can lead to fluid retention, electrolyte imbalances, and peripheral edema. Edema may be present in patients with oliguric or anuric AKI and signs of volume overload on physical examination.
2. **Chronic Kidney Disease (CKD):** CKD is associated with impaired renal function, electrolyte abnormalities, and fluid retention. Peripheral edema may be present in patients with advanced CKD and signs of volume overload, hypertension, or proteinuria.
3. **Nephrotic Syndrome:** Nephrotic syndrome, characterized by proteinuria, hypoalbuminemia, hyperlipidemia, and peripheral edema, may result from glomerular diseases such as minimal change disease, focal segmental glomerulosclerosis, or

membranous nephropathy.

Hepatic Dysfunction:

Hepatic dysfunction can lead to fluid retention and peripheral edema and may include:

1. **Cirrhosis:** Cirrhosis is associated with portal hypertension, hypoalbuminemia, and fluid retention, leading to ascites, peripheral edema, and hepatorenal syndrome. Clinical features of cirrhosis-related edema may include abdominal distension, lower extremity edema, and signs of hepatic decompensation.
2. **Congestive Hepatopathy:** Congestive hepatopathy, secondary to right-sided heart failure or hepatic venous outflow obstruction, can result in hepatic congestion, portal hypertension, and peripheral edema. Edema may be present in patients with signs of congestive hepatopathy and hepatic dysfunction.

Venous Insufficiency:

Venous insufficiency is a common cause of peripheral edema and may include:

1. **Chronic Venous Insufficiency (CVI):** CVI is characterized by impaired venous return, venous hypertension, and fluid extravasation into the interstitial spaces. Peripheral edema may be present in patients with CVI, particularly in the lower extremities, associated with venous stasis ulcers, varicose veins, or venous eczema.
2. **Deep Vein Thrombosis (DVT):** DVT, characterized by thrombus formation in the deep veins of the lower extremities, can lead to venous obstruction, venous reflux, and peripheral edema. Edema may be unilateral in patients with DVT and associated with pain,

swelling, and erythema.

Lymphatic Disorders:

Lymphatic disorders can lead to lymphedema, characterized by impaired lymphatic drainage and tissue swelling, and may include:

1. **Primary Lymphedema:** Primary lymphedema, often congenital or hereditary in nature, results from developmental abnormalities or genetic mutations affecting the lymphatic system. Peripheral edema may be present in patients with primary lymphedema, typically involving one or more extremities and associated with lymphatic dysfunction.
2. **Secondary Lymphedema:** Secondary lymphedema occurs due to acquired damage or obstruction of the lymphatic system, secondary to surgery, radiation therapy, trauma, infection, or malignancy. Edema may be localized or generalized in patients with secondary lymphedema, depending on the underlying cause and extent of lymphatic impairment.

Inflammatory Conditions:

Inflammatory conditions can lead to edema formation and may include:

1. **Inflammatory Bowel Disease (IBD):** IBD, including Crohn's disease and ulcerative colitis, can lead to protein-losing enteropathy, malabsorption, and peripheral edema. Edema may be present in patients with active IBD, particularly in the setting of hypoalbuminemia and protein loss.
2. **Rheumatoid Arthritis (RA):** RA is associated with systemic inflammation, synovitis, and joint effusions, which can lead to peripheral edema and swelling.

Edema may be present in patients with active RA, particularly in the hands, wrists, and ankles, associated with joint inflammation and effusion.

Endocrine Disorders:

Endocrine disorders can lead to fluid imbalance and peripheral edema and may include:

1. **Hypothyroidism:** Hypothyroidism is associated with reduced metabolic rate, fluid retention, and peripheral edema. Edema may be present in patients with hypothyroidism, particularly in the face, hands, and lower extremities, associated with myxedema and non-pitting edema.
2. **Cushing's Syndrome:** Cushing's syndrome, characterized by excessive cortisol production, sodium retention, and fluid overload, can lead to peripheral edema and weight gain. Edema may be present in patients with Cushing's syndrome, particularly in the face, trunk, and proximal extremities, associated with central obesity and striae.

Medication-Related Adverse Effects:

Medications can lead to fluid retention and peripheral edema as an adverse effect and may include:

1. **Calcium Channel Blockers:** Calcium channel blockers, such as amlodipine or nifedipine, can lead to peripheral edema due to vasodilation and increased capillary permeability.
2. **Nonsteroidal Anti-Inflammatory Drugs (NSAIDs):** NSAIDs, such as ibuprofen or naproxen, can lead to peripheral edema due to sodium retention and decreased renal blood flow.

Less Common Etiologies:

Less common etiologies of edema may include:

1. **Malnutrition:** Malnutrition, particularly protein-energy malnutrition, can lead to hypoalbuminemia, fluid retention, and peripheral edema. Edema may be present in patients with severe malnutrition, associated with wasting, cachexia, and nutritional deficiencies.
2. **Infections:** Infectious diseases, such as cellulitis, abscesses, or sepsis, can lead to localized or generalized edema secondary to inflammation, tissue damage, or septic shock.
3. **Malignancy:** Malignant tumors, particularly solid tumors or lymphomas, can lead to localized or systemic edema secondary to lymphatic obstruction, tumor invasion, or paraneoplastic syndromes.

Conclusion:

In conclusion, the differential diagnosis of edema encompasses a broad range of medical conditions that can lead to fluid accumulation in the interstitial spaces of tissues. Cardiovascular disorders, renal diseases, hepatic dysfunction, venous insufficiency, lymphatic disorders, inflammatory conditions, endocrine disorders, medication-related adverse effects, and other less common etiologies may contribute to the development of edema. A systematic approach to diagnostic evaluation, including comprehensive history-taking, physical examination, laboratory tests, and imaging studies, is essential for identifying the underlying cause of edema and guiding appropriate management strategies. Early recognition, timely intervention, and multidisciplinary collaboration are essential for optimizing patient care and improving clinical outcomes in patients with edema-related disorders.

CHAPTER 6: MANAGEMENT AND TREATMENT APPROACHES

Lifestyle Modifications and Dietary Management for Edema: Empowering Patients for Holistic Health

Edema, characterized by the abnormal accumulation of fluid in the interstitial spaces of tissues, often necessitates a multifaceted approach to management that includes lifestyle modifications and dietary interventions. Lifestyle modifications encompass a range of behavioral changes aimed at addressing underlying risk factors, promoting fluid balance, and optimizing overall health and well-being. Similarly, dietary management plays a pivotal role in edema management by regulating fluid intake, sodium consumption, protein intake, and micronutrient supplementation. This exploration delves into the principles of lifestyle modifications and dietary management for edema, providing insights into holistic approaches to empower patients in their journey towards optimal health.

Lifestyle Modifications:

1. **Regular Physical Activity:** Engaging in regular physical activity is essential for promoting cardiovascular health, enhancing lymphatic circulation, and reducing fluid retention. Aerobic exercises, such as walking, swimming, cycling, or low-impact aerobics, can help improve venous return, lymphatic drainage, and overall circulation, thereby reducing the risk of edema formation.
2. **Maintaining Healthy Body Weight:** Maintaining a healthy body weight is important for reducing the risk of obesity-related edema and metabolic complications. Adopting a balanced diet, incorporating regular physical activity, and practicing portion control can help achieve and maintain a healthy weight, thereby mitigating the burden of excess adiposity on cardiovascular and lymphatic function.
3. **Elevating Lower Extremities:** Elevating the lower extremities above heart level can help reduce dependent edema and improve venous return. Encouraging patients to elevate their legs while resting or sleeping can facilitate drainage of excess fluid from the lower limbs, alleviate discomfort, and promote lymphatic circulation.
4. **Avoiding Prolonged Sitting or Standing:** Prolonged sitting or standing can impede venous return, exacerbate venous insufficiency, and contribute to fluid accumulation in the lower extremities. Encouraging regular movement, periodic leg exercises, and avoiding prolonged periods of immobility can help prevent venous stasis and reduce the risk of edema formation.
5. **Compression Therapy:** Compression therapy involves

the use of compression garments, such as elastic stockings or bandages, to apply external pressure to the limbs and promote venous return. Compression therapy can help reduce peripheral edema, prevent venous pooling, and alleviate symptoms of venous insufficiency, particularly in patients with chronic venous disorders.
6. **Limb Elevation:** Elevating the affected limb above heart level can facilitate drainage of excess fluid from the interstitial spaces, reduce tissue congestion, and alleviate symptoms of peripheral edema. Encouraging patients to elevate their limbs regularly throughout the day, particularly during periods of rest or sleep, can help minimize dependent edema and improve lymphatic drainage.

Dietary Management:

1. **Sodium Restriction:** Sodium restriction is a cornerstone of dietary management for edema, as excessive sodium intake can lead to fluid retention, volume overload, and exacerbation of edema. Encouraging patients to reduce their intake of high-sodium foods, such as processed foods, canned soups, salty snacks, and fast food, can help mitigate sodium-induced fluid retention and promote fluid balance.
2. **Fluid Restriction:** Fluid restriction may be recommended in patients with severe edema or fluid overload, particularly in the setting of congestive heart failure or renal dysfunction. Monitoring fluid intake, limiting intake of high-volume beverages such as soda, juice, and caffeinated beverages, and practicing portion control during meals can help prevent excessive fluid intake and reduce the risk of volume overload.
3. **Potassium-Rich Foods:** Consuming potassium-rich

foods, such as fruits, vegetables, legumes, and dairy products, can help counteract the effects of sodium on fluid balance and promote diuresis. Encouraging patients to incorporate potassium-rich foods into their diet can help maintain electrolyte balance, reduce fluid retention, and support cardiovascular health.

4. **Protein Intake:** Adequate protein intake is essential for maintaining oncotic pressure, supporting tissue repair, and preserving lean body mass in patients with edema. Encouraging patients to consume lean sources of protein, such as poultry, fish, eggs, tofu, and legumes, can help optimize protein intake and mitigate the risk of hypoalbuminemia-related edema.

5. **Micronutrient Supplementation:** Micronutrient supplementation, including vitamins and minerals such as vitamin C, vitamin E, magnesium, and zinc, may be beneficial in supporting vascular health, reducing oxidative stress, and promoting lymphatic function. Encouraging patients to incorporate nutrient-rich foods into their diet or consider supplementation under the guidance of a healthcare professional can help optimize micronutrient status and support edema management.

6. **Fluid Monitoring:** Monitoring fluid intake and output can help patients maintain fluid balance and prevent excessive fluid retention. Encouraging patients to track their fluid intake, monitor urine output, and adjust their fluid intake based on individual needs, hydration status, and clinical recommendations can help optimize fluid balance and prevent volume overload.

Conclusion:

In conclusion, lifestyle modifications and dietary management play a pivotal role in the management of edema by addressing underlying risk factors, promoting fluid balance, and optimizing overall health and well-being. Adopting a holistic approach that encompasses regular physical activity, maintaining a healthy body weight, elevating lower extremities, avoiding prolonged sitting or standing, and incorporating compression therapy can help reduce the risk of edema formation and alleviate symptoms of peripheral edema. Similarly, dietary modifications such as sodium restriction, fluid restriction, consumption of potassium-rich foods, adequate protein intake, micronutrient supplementation, and fluid monitoring can help optimize fluid balance, support cardiovascular health, and mitigate the burden of edema-related complications. Empowering patients with knowledge, resources, and support to implement lifestyle modifications and dietary interventions is essential for promoting self-management, enhancing quality of life, and achieving optimal outcomes in patients with edema. By embracing a holistic approach that addresses the multifaceted nature of edema, healthcare providers can empower patients to take an active role in their care and embark on a journey towards holistic health and well-being.

Pharmacological Interventions for Edema: Exploring Diuretics, Vasodilators, and Anti-inflammatory Agents

Pharmacological interventions play a crucial role in the management of edema by targeting underlying mechanisms of fluid retention, volume overload, and inflammation. Diuretics, vasodilators, and anti-inflammatory agents represent key classes of medications used in the treatment of edema, each exerting distinct mechanisms of action to alleviate symptoms, improve fluid balance, and optimize patient outcomes. This exploration delves into the pharmacological interventions for edema, encompassing diuretics, vasodilators, and anti-inflammatory agents, providing insights into their mechanisms of action, indications, adverse effects, and clinical considerations in the management of fluid imbalance disorders.

Diuretics:

Diuretics are a cornerstone of pharmacological therapy for edema and work by increasing renal excretion of sodium and water, thereby reducing extracellular fluid volume and alleviating symptoms of fluid overload. Commonly used diuretics in the management of edema include:

1. **Thiazide Diuretics:** Thiazide diuretics, such as hydrochlorothiazide and chlorthalidone, inhibit sodium reabsorption in the distal convoluted tubule of the nephron, leading to increased sodium and water excretion. Thiazide diuretics are effective in the treatment of mild to moderate edema and are often used as first-line agents in patients with hypertension and volume overload.
2. **Loop Diuretics:** Loop diuretics, such as furosemide, bumetanide, and torsemide, inhibit sodium reabsorption in the thick ascending limb of the loop of Henle, leading to profound diuresis and natriuresis. Loop diuretics are potent agents used in the management of severe edema associated with heart failure, renal failure, and liver cirrhosis, as well as acute pulmonary edema.
3. **Potassium-Sparing Diuretics:** Potassium-sparing diuretics, such as spironolactone, eplerenone, and amiloride, exert their diuretic effects by antagonizing the actions of aldosterone, thereby promoting sodium excretion and potassium retention. Potassium-sparing diuretics are often used as adjunctive therapy in

patients with refractory edema or as a means of preventing hypokalemia associated with loop or thiazide diuretic therapy.

Vasodilators:

Vasodilators are medications that dilate blood vessels, thereby reducing venous pressure, improving venous return, and alleviating symptoms of peripheral edema. Commonly used vasodilators in the management of edema include:

1. **Calcium Channel Blockers:** Calcium channel blockers, such as amlodipine, nifedipine, and diltiazem, inhibit calcium influx into vascular smooth muscle cells, leading to relaxation of arterial and venous smooth muscle and vasodilation. Calcium channel blockers are effective in the treatment of hypertension, angina, and peripheral vascular disease and may be used adjunctively in patients with edema associated with venous insufficiency or arterial vasospasm.
2. **Nitrates:** Nitrates, such as nitroglycerin and isosorbide dinitrate, release nitric oxide, a potent vasodilator, which relaxes vascular smooth muscle and dilates blood vessels. Nitrates are used in the management of angina, acute coronary syndromes, and congestive heart failure, where they can help reduce preload, improve cardiac output, and alleviate symptoms of pulmonary and peripheral edema.
3. **Hydralazine:** Hydralazine is a direct-acting arterial vasodilator that relaxes vascular smooth muscle and reduces systemic vascular resistance. Hydralazine is used in the treatment of hypertension, particularly in patients with severe hypertension or hypertensive emergencies, where it can help reduce afterload, improve cardiac output, and mitigate symptoms of volume overload and pulmonary congestion.

Anti-inflammatory Agents:

Inflammation plays a pivotal role in the pathogenesis of edema, particularly in conditions associated with tissue injury, endothelial dysfunction, and capillary leakage. Anti-inflammatory agents target inflammatory pathways and mediators to reduce tissue inflammation, endothelial permeability, and fluid extravasation. Commonly used anti-inflammatory agents in the management of edema include:

1. **Nonsteroidal Anti-inflammatory Drugs (NSAIDs):** NSAIDs, such as ibuprofen, naproxen, and diclofenac, inhibit cyclooxygenase enzymes and prostaglandin synthesis, thereby reducing inflammation, pain, and swelling. NSAIDs are used in the treatment of inflammatory conditions, such as arthritis, tendonitis, and bursitis, where they can help alleviate symptoms of localized edema and tissue inflammation.
2. **Corticosteroids:** Corticosteroids, such as prednisone, dexamethasone, and methylprednisolone, exert potent anti-inflammatory effects by suppressing immune responses, cytokine production, and inflammatory signaling pathways. Corticosteroids are used in the treatment of inflammatory conditions, autoimmune diseases, and allergic reactions, where they can help reduce tissue inflammation, edema formation, and immune-mediated tissue damage.
3. **Biological Agents:** Biological agents, such as tumor necrosis factor-alpha (TNF-alpha) inhibitors, interleukin-1 (IL-1) inhibitors, and monoclonal antibodies, target specific inflammatory cytokines and pathways involved in the pathogenesis of inflammatory disorders. Biological agents are used in the treatment of autoimmune diseases, inflammatory bowel disease, and rheumatic conditions, where they

can help suppress inflammatory responses, reduce tissue edema, and improve clinical outcomes.

Clinical Considerations:

1. **Individualized Therapy:** Pharmacological management of edema should be individualized based on the underlying etiology, severity of symptoms, comorbidities, and patient preferences. A thorough clinical assessment, including medical history, physical examination, and diagnostic evaluation, is essential for determining the appropriate pharmacological interventions and optimizing treatment outcomes.
2. **Monitoring and Titration:** Regular monitoring of clinical symptoms, fluid status, electrolyte levels, renal function, and adverse effects is essential during pharmacological therapy for edema. Titration of medication dosages, adjustment of treatment regimens, and consideration of combination therapy may be necessary to achieve optimal fluid balance, symptom relief, and therapeutic efficacy.
3. **Adverse Effects:** Pharmacological agents used in the management of edema may be associated with adverse effects, including electrolyte imbalances, hypotension, renal dysfunction, gastrointestinal disturbances, and drug interactions. Healthcare providers should be vigilant for signs of adverse effects and provide appropriate monitoring, counseling, and supportive care to minimize risks and optimize patient safety.
4. **Multidisciplinary Approach:** The management of edema often requires a multidisciplinary approach involving collaboration between primary care providers, cardiologists, nephrologists, hepatologists, vascular specialists, and allied healthcare professionals. Multidisciplinary teams can facilitate

comprehensive assessment, individualized treatment planning, and coordinated care delivery to optimize patient outcomes and improve quality of life.

Conclusion:

In conclusion, pharmacological interventions play a pivotal role in the management of edema by targeting underlying mechanisms of fluid retention, volume overload, and inflammation. Diuretics, vasodilators, and anti-inflammatory agents represent key classes of medications used in the treatment of edema, each exerting distinct mechanisms of action to alleviate symptoms, improve fluid balance, and optimize patient outcomes. Individualized therapy, regular monitoring, consideration of adverse effects, and multidisciplinary collaboration are essential components of pharmacological management for edema, ensuring safe and effective treatment strategies tailored to the needs of each patient. By embracing a comprehensive approach that integrates pharmacological interventions with lifestyle modifications, dietary management, and supportive care, healthcare providers can empower patients in their journey towards optimal fluid balance, symptom relief, and holistic health.

Non-pharmacological Interventions for Edema: Embracing Compression Therapy, Elevation, and Physical Therapy

Edema, characterized by the abnormal accumulation of fluid in the interstitial spaces of tissues, often requires a comprehensive approach to management that includes non-pharmacological interventions aimed at reducing fluid retention, improving lymphatic circulation, and alleviating symptoms of peripheral swelling. Non-pharmacological interventions play a pivotal role in the management of edema by complementing pharmacological therapy, promoting self-management, and optimizing patient outcomes. This exploration delves into the non-pharmacological interventions for edema, encompassing compression therapy, elevation, physical therapy, and lifestyle modifications, providing insights into their mechanisms of action, indications, clinical applications, and evidence-based practices in the management of fluid imbalance disorders.

Compression Therapy:

Compression therapy involves the application of external pressure to the limbs using compression garments, bandages, or pneumatic devices to promote venous return, reduce venous hypertension, and alleviate symptoms of peripheral edema. Commonly used compression modalities in the management of edema include:

1. **Compression Stockings:** Compression stockings, also known as support hose or compression socks, are elastic garments worn on the lower extremities to exert graduated compression, with maximum pressure at the ankle and decreasing pressure towards the thigh or knee. Compression stockings help improve venous return, prevent venous pooling, and reduce edema formation in patients with chronic venous insufficiency, varicose veins, or lymphatic disorders.

2. **Compression Bandages:** Compression bandages are elastic or inelastic wraps applied to the limbs to provide circumferential compression and support. Short-stretch bandages, such as cohesive bandages or multi-layer compression wraps, are commonly used in the treatment of venous ulcers, lymphedema, and postoperative edema to reduce tissue swelling, promote lymphatic drainage, and facilitate wound

healing.
3. **Intermittent Pneumatic Compression (IPC):** Intermittent pneumatic compression devices consist of inflatable sleeves or cuffs worn on the limbs that sequentially inflate and deflate to promote venous return and lymphatic drainage. IPC is used in the management of lymphedema, deep vein thrombosis (DVT), and venous insufficiency to reduce edema, prevent thrombosis, and improve circulation, particularly in patients with impaired mobility or venous stasis.

Elevation:

Elevation of the affected limb above heart level is a simple yet effective non-pharmacological intervention for reducing dependent edema, improving lymphatic drainage, and alleviating symptoms of peripheral swelling. Elevation works by reducing hydrostatic pressure in the veins, promoting venous return, and facilitating fluid drainage from the interstitial spaces. Key principles of limb elevation in the management of edema include:

1. **Supine Position:** Patients are advised to lie down in a supine position with the affected limb elevated above heart level, using pillows or cushions to support the limb and maintain elevation. Supine elevation facilitates venous return from the lower extremities, reduces venous pooling, and minimizes dependent edema in patients with peripheral swelling.
2. **Regular Elevation:** Patients are encouraged to elevate the affected limb regularly throughout the day, particularly during periods of rest or sleep, to promote continuous drainage of excess fluid and prevent fluid accumulation. Regular elevation helps mitigate symptoms of edema, improve tissue perfusion,

and enhance lymphatic circulation in patients with chronic venous insufficiency or lymphatic dysfunction.

3. **Activity Modification:** Patients are instructed to avoid prolonged standing or sitting and engage in periodic leg elevation breaks to prevent venous stasis, reduce tissue congestion, and minimize the risk of edema formation. Activity modification, including frequent changes in position, ambulation, and leg exercises, can help optimize venous return and lymphatic drainage in patients with venous or lymphatic disorders.

Physical Therapy:

Physical therapy plays a vital role in the management of edema by promoting mobility, muscle pump function, and lymphatic drainage through therapeutic exercises, manual techniques, and patient education. Key components of physical therapy for edema management include:

1. **Manual Lymphatic Drainage (MLD):** MLD is a specialized massage technique performed by trained therapists to stimulate lymphatic vessels, enhance lymphatic flow, and reduce tissue swelling. MLD involves gentle, rhythmic strokes applied to the skin in specific patterns to promote lymphatic drainage and alleviate symptoms of lymphedema, postoperative edema, or venous insufficiency.

2. **Compression Therapy:** Physical therapists may prescribe compression garments, bandages, or pneumatic devices to augment the effects of manual lymphatic drainage and promote sustained reduction in tissue swelling. Compression therapy helps maintain gains achieved through MLD, prevent re-accumulation of fluid, and support ongoing management of chronic edema conditions.

3. **Exercise Prescription:** Exercise prescription tailored to the individual patient's needs, functional abilities, and clinical status can help improve muscle pump function, enhance venous return, and facilitate lymphatic drainage. Therapeutic exercises, such as ankle pumps, calf raises, leg cycling, and walking, can help activate muscle contraction, increase blood flow, and reduce edema formation in patients with peripheral swelling.
4. **Education and Self-management:** Physical therapists provide education on edema management strategies, including skin care, hygiene, compression garment application, exercise adherence, and lifestyle modifications. Empowering patients with knowledge, skills, and self-management techniques can help promote independence, adherence to treatment, and long-term success in managing edema-related symptoms and complications.

Clinical Considerations:

1. **Individualized Treatment:** Non-pharmacological interventions for edema should be individualized based on the underlying etiology, severity of symptoms, patient preferences, and functional status. A comprehensive assessment, including clinical evaluation, diagnostic testing, and multidisciplinary consultation, is essential for determining the most appropriate non-pharmacological interventions and optimizing treatment outcomes.
2. **Combination Therapy:** Non-pharmacological interventions are often used in combination with pharmacological therapy, lifestyle modifications, and other treatment modalities to achieve optimal fluid balance, symptom relief, and functional improvement. Combining compression therapy, elevation, and

physical therapy techniques can synergistically enhance lymphatic drainage, reduce tissue swelling, and improve patient outcomes in the management of edema.

3. **Adherence and Compliance:** Adherence to non-pharmacological interventions requires patient education, support, and ongoing reinforcement to ensure compliance with treatment recommendations. Healthcare providers should engage patients in shared decision-making, address barriers to adherence, and provide resources for self-management to enhance treatment adherence and optimize long-term outcomes in patients with edema.

Conclusion:

In conclusion, non-pharmacological interventions play a pivotal role in the management of edema by reducing fluid retention, improving lymphatic circulation, and alleviating symptoms of peripheral swelling. Compression therapy, elevation, physical therapy, and lifestyle modifications are integral components of holistic edema management, offering safe, effective, and patient-centered approaches to optimizing fluid balance and improving quality of life. Individualized treatment, combination therapy, and adherence to treatment recommendations are essential considerations in the implementation of non-pharmacological interventions for edema, ensuring comprehensive care and favorable outcomes in patients with fluid imbalance disorders. By embracing a multidisciplinary approach that integrates non-pharmacological interventions with pharmacological therapy, patient education, and supportive care, healthcare providers can empower patients to take an active role in their edema management and achieve optimal health and well-being.

Surgical Interventions for Edema: Exploring Lymphatic Surgery and Vascular Procedures

In cases where conservative measures and pharmacological interventions prove insufficient in managing edema, surgical interventions may offer viable solutions to address underlying anatomical or functional abnormalities contributing to fluid imbalance. Surgical approaches for edema encompass a spectrum of procedures aimed at improving lymphatic drainage, restoring venous function, and alleviating symptoms of peripheral swelling. This exploration delves into surgical interventions for edema, focusing on lymphatic surgery and vascular procedures, providing insights into their indications, techniques, outcomes, and considerations in the management of fluid imbalance disorders.

Lymphatic Surgery:

Lymphatic surgery encompasses a range of procedures aimed at improving lymphatic drainage, reducing tissue swelling, and alleviating symptoms of lymphedema, a chronic condition characterized by impaired lymphatic function and persistent fluid accumulation. Commonly used lymphatic surgery techniques include:

1. **Lymphovenous Anastomosis (LVA):** Lymphovenous anastomosis involves the direct connection of lymphatic vessels to adjacent veins to bypass obstructed or damaged lymphatic channels and facilitate lymphatic drainage. LVA is performed using microsurgical techniques and specialized instruments to create small lymphaticovenous shunts, allowing

lymphatic fluid to enter the venous system and reduce tissue swelling. LVA is indicated in patients with early-stage lymphedema and suitable lymphatic vessels amenable to surgical intervention.

2. **Vascularized Lymph Node Transfer (VLNT):** Vascularized lymph node transfer involves the microsurgical transplantation of lymph nodes from a donor site to the affected limb to restore lymphatic function, improve lymphatic drainage, and reduce tissue swelling. VLNT utilizes autologous tissue grafts, typically harvested from the groin or abdomen, to provide a source of healthy lymphatic tissue and lymphatic vessels for reconstruction. VLNT is indicated in patients with advanced-stage lymphedema or inadequate response to conservative therapy, where surgical revascularization of lymphatic tissue is warranted.

3. **Lymphaticovenous Bypass (LVB):** Lymphaticovenous bypass involves the creation of direct connections between lymphatic vessels and adjacent veins using microsurgical techniques to divert lymphatic fluid away from congested areas and promote venous return. LVB is indicated in patients with localized lymphedema, such as secondary lymphedema following cancer treatment or trauma, where targeted surgical intervention can alleviate tissue swelling and improve lymphatic function.

4. **Liposuction:** Liposuction is a surgical procedure that involves the removal of excess adipose tissue from subcutaneous compartments to reduce tissue volume and alleviate symptoms of lymphedema. Liposuction is used as an adjunctive therapy in patients with fibroadipose tissue deposition and refractory lymphedema, where conservative measures and lymphatic surgery may not provide adequate relief.

Liposuction techniques, such as tumescent liposuction or power-assisted liposuction, are employed to minimize trauma and optimize aesthetic outcomes.

Vascular Procedures:

Vascular procedures for edema encompass interventions aimed at restoring venous function, improving venous return, and reducing venous hypertension to alleviate symptoms of peripheral swelling. Commonly used vascular procedures in the management of edema include:

1. **Venous Valve Repair or Reconstruction:** Venous valve repair or reconstruction involves surgical repair or replacement of damaged or incompetent venous valves to restore normal venous function, prevent venous reflux, and improve venous return. Venous valve repair techniques, such as valvuloplasty or neovalve creation, are performed using microsurgical techniques to enhance venous hemodynamics and alleviate symptoms of chronic venous insufficiency.
2. **Venous Bypass Surgery:** Venous bypass surgery involves the creation of alternative venous pathways to bypass obstructed or incompetent veins and restore venous drainage. Venous bypass techniques, such as vein grafting or venous interposition, are employed to reroute blood flow around diseased segments of veins and alleviate symptoms of venous obstruction, such as limb swelling, pain, and skin changes.
3. **Venous Stenting:** Venous stenting involves the placement of endovascular stents within obstructed or compressed veins to restore luminal patency, improve venous flow, and alleviate symptoms of venous congestion. Venous stenting is indicated in patients with venous stenosis, thrombosis, or compression syndromes, such as May-Thurner syndrome or iliac

vein compression, where surgical intervention is warranted to optimize venous hemodynamics and prevent recurrent edema.

4. **Venous Thrombectomy:** Venous thrombectomy involves the surgical removal of thrombi or emboli from obstructed veins to restore venous patency, prevent venous occlusion, and alleviate symptoms of acute or chronic venous insufficiency. Venous thrombectomy techniques, such as open thrombectomy or catheter-directed thrombolysis, are employed to remove obstructing thrombus and restore venous flow in patients with acute deep vein thrombosis (DVT) or chronic venous occlusive disease.

Clinical Considerations:

1. **Patient Selection:** Surgical interventions for edema should be carefully considered and individualized based on patient characteristics, disease severity, anatomical considerations, and treatment goals. A comprehensive evaluation, including clinical assessment, imaging studies, lymphatic mapping, and functional testing, is essential for selecting appropriate candidates for surgical intervention and optimizing treatment outcomes.

2. **Multidisciplinary Collaboration:** Surgical management of edema often requires multidisciplinary collaboration between surgeons, interventional radiologists, lymphedema therapists, and allied healthcare professionals to ensure comprehensive assessment, perioperative care, and long-term follow-up. Multidisciplinary teams can provide expert guidance, coordinate treatment planning, and optimize patient care throughout the surgical journey.

3. **Preoperative Preparation:** Preoperative preparation

for surgical interventions for edema involves optimizing patient health, addressing comorbidities, and mitigating risk factors to minimize perioperative complications and enhance surgical outcomes. Preoperative assessment, medical optimization, nutritional support, and psychological counseling are essential components of preoperative care in patients undergoing lymphatic surgery or vascular procedures for edema.

4. **Postoperative Management:** Postoperative management following surgical interventions for edema involves close monitoring, wound care, compression therapy, and rehabilitation to facilitate recovery, optimize lymphatic function, and prevent complications. Postoperative surveillance, lymphedema therapy, and long-term follow-up are essential for monitoring treatment response, assessing outcomes, and addressing any postoperative issues that may arise.

Conclusion:

In conclusion, surgical interventions play a crucial role in the management of edema by addressing underlying anatomical or functional abnormalities contributing to fluid imbalance. Lymphatic surgery and vascular procedures offer viable options for improving lymphatic drainage, restoring venous function, and alleviating symptoms of peripheral swelling in patients with lymphedema, chronic venous insufficiency, or other fluid imbalance disorders. Patient selection, multidisciplinary collaboration, preoperative preparation, and postoperative management are essential considerations in the implementation of surgical interventions for edema, ensuring safe, effective, and patient-centered care. By embracing a comprehensive approach that integrates surgical interventions with conservative measures, pharmacological therapy, and supportive care, healthcare providers can optimize treatment outcomes and improve quality of life for patients with fluid imbalance disorders.

Management of Underlying Conditions Contributing to Edema: A Comprehensive Approach

Edema, characterized by the abnormal accumulation of fluid in the interstitial spaces of tissues, often arises as a manifestation of underlying conditions that disrupt fluid balance, impair lymphatic function, or compromise venous circulation. Effective management of edema necessitates a comprehensive approach that addresses the underlying etiology, treats associated comorbidities, and mitigates risk factors contributing to fluid imbalance. This exploration delves into the management of underlying conditions contributing to edema, encompassing cardiovascular disorders, renal dysfunction, liver disease, lymphatic disorders, and systemic conditions, providing insights into diagnostic strategies, treatment modalities, and holistic approaches to optimize patient outcomes.

Cardiovascular Disorders:

1. **Congestive Heart Failure (CHF):** Management of edema in patients with CHF focuses on optimizing cardiac function, reducing fluid retention, and alleviating symptoms of volume overload. Treatment strategies include diuretic therapy to promote diuresis, sodium restriction to minimize fluid retention, and pharmacological agents such as angiotensin-converting enzyme (ACE) inhibitors or angiotensin II receptor blockers (ARBs) to improve cardiac function and reduce venous congestion.

2. **Chronic Venous Insufficiency (CVI):** Management of edema in patients with CVI aims to improve venous circulation, reduce venous hypertension, and alleviate symptoms of peripheral swelling. Treatment modalities include compression therapy with compression stockings or bandages, elevation of the affected limb to promote venous return, and venous interventions such as venous ablation or sclerotherapy to address underlying venous reflux or obstruction.

Renal Dysfunction:

1. **Nephrotic Syndrome:** Management of edema in patients with nephrotic syndrome involves treating the underlying renal pathology, reducing proteinuria, and optimizing fluid balance. Treatment modalities include corticosteroids or immunosuppressive agents to control disease activity, angiotensin-converting enzyme inhibitors (ACEIs) or angiotensin II receptor blockers (ARBs) to reduce proteinuria, and diuretic therapy to promote diuresis and alleviate fluid retention.
2. **Acute Kidney Injury (AKI):** Management of edema in patients with AKI focuses on addressing the underlying cause of renal dysfunction, optimizing fluid status, and preventing complications such as volume overload or electrolyte imbalances. Treatment strategies include fluid restriction to prevent fluid overload, diuretic therapy to promote diuresis and maintain fluid balance, and renal replacement therapy (e.g., hemodialysis or continuous renal replacement therapy) in severe cases of AKI.

Liver Disease:

1. **Cirrhosis:** Management of edema in patients with

cirrhosis involves addressing portal hypertension, reducing ascites formation, and improving hepatic function. Treatment modalities include sodium restriction to minimize fluid retention, diuretic therapy (e.g., spironolactone or furosemide) to promote diuresis and reduce ascites, and procedures such as paracentesis or transjugular intrahepatic portosystemic shunt (TIPS) placement in refractory cases of ascites.

2. **Portal Hypertension:** Management of edema in patients with portal hypertension focuses on reducing portal pressure, preventing variceal bleeding, and minimizing complications such as ascites or hepatic encephalopathy. Treatment strategies include beta-blockers to reduce portal pressure, endoscopic variceal ligation (EVL) or sclerotherapy to prevent variceal bleeding, and procedures such as TIPS placement to decompress the portal system and alleviate ascites.

Lymphatic Disorders:

1. **Primary Lymphedema:** Management of edema in patients with primary lymphedema involves conservative measures, lymphatic drainage techniques, and supportive care to minimize tissue swelling and improve lymphatic function. Treatment modalities include manual lymphatic drainage (MLD) to stimulate lymphatic flow, compression therapy with compression garments or bandages to reduce limb swelling, and skincare to prevent complications such as cellulitis or lymphangitis.

2. **Secondary Lymphedema:** Management of edema in patients with secondary lymphedema focuses on treating the underlying cause of lymphatic obstruction or damage, reducing tissue swelling, and preventing recurrent episodes of lymphedema.

Treatment strategies include surgical interventions such as lymphovenous anastomosis (LVA) or vascularized lymph node transfer (VLNT) to restore lymphatic function, compression therapy to alleviate limb swelling, and physical therapy to promote lymphatic drainage and improve functional outcomes.

Systemic Conditions:

1. **Hypoproteinemia:** Management of edema in patients with hypoproteinemia involves addressing the underlying protein deficiency, optimizing nutritional status, and preventing complications such as hypoalbuminemia-related edema. Treatment modalities include dietary protein supplementation to correct protein deficiency, nutritional support to improve protein intake and absorption, and pharmacological agents such as albumin infusions to restore serum albumin levels and reduce fluid retention.
2. **Inflammatory Disorders:** Management of edema in patients with inflammatory disorders focuses on controlling inflammation, reducing tissue edema, and alleviating symptoms of peripheral swelling. Treatment strategies include anti-inflammatory medications such as nonsteroidal anti-inflammatory drugs (NSAIDs) or corticosteroids to suppress inflammatory responses, disease-modifying antirheumatic drugs (DMARDs) to control autoimmune disease activity, and lifestyle modifications to minimize exacerbating factors such as dietary triggers or environmental allergens.

Holistic Approaches:

1. **Patient Education:** Empowering patients with

knowledge about their underlying condition, treatment options, and self-management strategies is essential for optimizing adherence, promoting self-care, and improving treatment outcomes. Patient education should encompass information about dietary modifications, medication adherence, symptom recognition, and when to seek medical attention for worsening symptoms or complications.
2. **Lifestyle Modifications:** Encouraging patients to adopt healthy lifestyle habits, including regular exercise, smoking cessation, stress management, and weight management, can help improve overall health, reduce inflammation, and optimize fluid balance. Lifestyle modifications such as sodium restriction, alcohol moderation, and hydration management can also complement pharmacological therapy and enhance treatment efficacy in managing edema-related conditions.

Conclusion:

In conclusion, the management of edema necessitates a comprehensive approach that addresses underlying conditions contributing to fluid imbalance, treats associated comorbidities, and mitigates risk factors to optimize patient outcomes. Management strategies for edema-associated conditions such as cardiovascular disorders, renal dysfunction, liver disease, lymphatic disorders, and systemic conditions encompass a spectrum of interventions ranging from pharmacological therapy and surgical interventions to lifestyle modifications and supportive care. By embracing a holistic approach that integrates diagnostic evaluation, personalized treatment planning, and patient-centered care, healthcare providers can effectively manage underlying conditions contributing to edema, alleviate symptoms of peripheral swelling, and improve quality of life for patients with fluid imbalance disorders.

CHAPTER 7: COMPLICATIONS AND PROGNOSIS

Complications Associated with Chronic Edema: Understanding Risks and Management Strategies

Chronic edema, characterized by persistent swelling due to the accumulation of fluid in the interstitial spaces of tissues, can lead to various complications that impact physical, psychological, and social well-being. Understanding the potential complications associated with chronic edema is crucial for healthcare providers to implement preventive measures, optimize treatment strategies, and improve patient outcomes. This exploration delves into the complications associated with chronic edema, encompassing skin changes, infections, impaired wound healing, functional limitations, and psychosocial impact, providing insights into their pathophysiology, clinical manifestations, and management strategies to mitigate risks and improve patient care.

Skin Changes:

1. **Skin Breakdown:** Chronic edema can lead to skin changes such as maceration, erythema, and breakdown, predisposing patients to the development of ulcers, wounds, and infections. Prolonged exposure to moisture, friction, and pressure in areas of edema can compromise skin integrity and increase the risk of tissue damage.
2. **Cellulitis:** Chronic edema is a significant risk factor for cellulitis, a bacterial infection of the skin and subcutaneous tissues characterized by erythema, warmth, swelling, and tenderness. Impaired lymphatic drainage and compromised skin barrier function in areas of edema create a favorable environment for bacterial colonization and infection.
3. **Lymphorrhea:** Lymphorrhea, or leakage of lymphatic fluid from the skin, can occur in patients with chronic edema, leading to maceration, excoriation, and secondary infection. Lymphorrhea is often observed in advanced cases of lymphedema or venous insufficiency, where impaired lymphatic drainage and compromised skin integrity contribute to fluid leakage.

Infections:

1. **Cellulitis:** Cellulitis is a common complication of chronic edema, particularly in patients with impaired lymphatic drainage or compromised skin barrier function. Prompt recognition and treatment of cellulitis are essential to prevent complications such as abscess formation, sepsis, and recurrent infections.
2. **Lymphangitis:** Lymphangitis, or inflammation of the lymphatic vessels, can occur secondary to bacterial invasion of the lymphatic system in patients with chronic edema. Lymphangitis presents with

symptoms such as red streaks, pain, swelling, and fever and may progress to systemic infection if left untreated.
3. **Abscess Formation:** Chronic edema increases the risk of abscess formation due to bacterial colonization of compromised tissue and impaired immune response. Abscesses may develop in areas of tissue breakdown, lymphatic stasis, or chronic inflammation and require prompt drainage and antibiotic therapy to prevent complications.

Impaired Wound Healing:

1. **Delayed Healing:** Chronic edema can impair wound healing by disrupting normal tissue repair processes, reducing tissue oxygenation, and impairing immune function. Prolonged inflammation, bacterial colonization, and tissue hypoxia in areas of edema contribute to delayed wound healing and increase the risk of complications such as infection and dehiscence.
2. **Chronic Wounds:** Chronic edema predisposes patients to the development of chronic wounds such as venous ulcers, arterial ulcers, and pressure ulcers, which are challenging to heal and prone to recurrence. Chronic wounds require comprehensive wound care, including debridement, dressings, offloading, and compression therapy, to promote healing and prevent complications.

Functional Limitations:

1. **Reduced Mobility:** Chronic edema can impair mobility and physical function due to pain, discomfort, and limitations in range of motion caused by tissue swelling and inflammation. Reduced mobility can lead to muscle weakness, joint stiffness, and functional

limitations, impacting activities of daily living and quality of life.
2. **Limb Disfigurement:** Severe chronic edema, such as lymphedema or advanced venous insufficiency, can cause limb disfigurement and deformity, leading to psychosocial distress and impaired body image. Limb disfigurement may result in social stigma, emotional distress, and reduced self-esteem, affecting interpersonal relationships and psychological well-being.

Psychosocial Impact:

1. **Depression and Anxiety:** Chronic edema can have a profound psychosocial impact, leading to feelings of depression, anxiety, and social isolation. The physical discomfort, functional limitations, and aesthetic concerns associated with chronic edema can negatively impact mental health and quality of life, exacerbating psychological distress and reducing overall well-being.
2. **Social Withdrawal:** Patients with chronic edema may experience social withdrawal and avoidance of social activities due to embarrassment, shame, or fear of stigma associated with their condition. Social isolation can exacerbate feelings of loneliness, depression, and anxiety, further compromising mental health and quality of life.

Management Strategies:

1. **Preventive Measures:** Preventive measures such as skincare, compression therapy, and lymphedema education are essential for reducing the risk of complications associated with chronic edema. Regular skincare, moisturization, and inspection of the skin

can help prevent skin breakdown, infections, and lymphorrhea.
2. **Early Recognition:** Early recognition of complications such as cellulitis, lymphangitis, or wound deterioration is crucial for prompt intervention and prevention of progression to severe infections or chronic wounds. Healthcare providers should educate patients about signs and symptoms of complications and encourage timely reporting and seeking medical attention.
3. **Comprehensive Wound Care:** Comprehensive wound care is essential for optimizing wound healing and preventing complications in patients with chronic edema-related wounds. This includes wound assessment, debridement, infection control, moisture management, and appropriate wound dressings tailored to the specific characteristics of the wound.
4. **Functional Rehabilitation:** Functional rehabilitation programs focused on mobility exercises, strength training, and adaptive strategies can help improve physical function and mobility in patients with chronic edema. Physical therapy interventions such as manual lymphatic drainage (MLD), therapeutic exercise, and compression therapy can enhance lymphatic drainage, reduce tissue swelling, and improve functional outcomes.
5. **Psychosocial Support:** Psychosocial support services such as counseling, support groups, and peer mentoring can help address the emotional and social challenges faced by patients with chronic edema. Providing emotional support, coping strategies, and resources for self-care can empower patients to manage their condition effectively and improve overall well-being.

Conclusion:

In conclusion, chronic edema is associated with various complications that impact physical health, wound healing, functional status, and psychosocial well-being. Understanding the potential complications of chronic edema is essential for healthcare providers to implement preventive measures, recognize early signs of complications, and optimize management strategies to improve patient outcomes. Comprehensive wound care, functional rehabilitation, psychosocial support, and patient education are essential components of holistic care for patients with chronic edema, aiming to mitigate risks, promote healing, and enhance quality of life. By adopting a multidisciplinary approach that addresses the complex needs of patients with chronic edema, healthcare providers can optimize treatment outcomes, prevent complications, and improve overall patient care and satisfaction.

Impact of Chronic Edema on Quality of Life and Functional Status: Understanding the Burden and Implementing Supportive Strategies

Chronic edema, characterized by persistent swelling due to fluid retention in the interstitial spaces of tissues, exerts a significant impact on the quality of life (QoL) and functional status of affected individuals. Understanding the multifaceted implications of chronic edema on physical, emotional, and social well-being is crucial for healthcare providers to implement supportive strategies, optimize treatment approaches, and improve overall patient outcomes. This exploration delves into the impact of chronic edema on quality of life and functional status, encompassing physical limitations, psychological distress, social implications, and practical challenges, providing insights into effective interventions and holistic approaches to enhance patient well-being and functional independence.

Physical Limitations:

1. **Reduced Mobility:** Chronic edema can lead to reduced mobility and physical function due to the heaviness, discomfort, and limitations in range of motion associated with tissue swelling. Patients may experience difficulty walking, standing, or performing activities of daily living, leading to functional impairment and dependence on caregivers for assistance.
2. **Functional Disability:** Severe chronic edema, such as lymphedema or advanced venous insufficiency, can cause functional disability and limitations in performing tasks requiring manual dexterity, such as dressing, grooming, and self-care. Edema-related symptoms such as pain, stiffness, and weakness can exacerbate functional limitations and impact overall independence and quality of life.

Psychological Distress:

1. **Anxiety and Depression:** Chronic edema can trigger feelings of anxiety, depression, and emotional distress due to the physical discomfort, body image concerns, and functional limitations associated with the condition. Patients may experience fear of exacerbations, social stigma, and uncertainty about the future, leading to heightened psychological distress and reduced mental well-being.
2. **Body Image Concerns:** Chronic edema-related

changes in body appearance, such as limb swelling, disfigurement, or skin changes, can negatively impact body image and self-esteem. Patients may experience embarrassment, shame, or social withdrawal due to perceived aesthetic flaws, further exacerbating psychological distress and impairing quality of life.

Social Implications:

1. **Social Isolation:** Chronic edema can lead to social isolation and withdrawal from social activities due to embarrassment, shame, or fear of stigma associated with visible swelling or disfigurement. Patients may avoid social gatherings, public places, or social interactions, leading to feelings of loneliness, isolation, and reduced social support.
2. **Impact on Relationships:** Chronic edema can strain interpersonal relationships and affect family dynamics, intimate relationships, and social interactions. Caregivers may experience increased burden, stress, and emotional strain in providing support and assistance to affected individuals, leading to caregiver fatigue and burnout.

Practical Challenges:

1. **Financial Burden:** Chronic edema-related medical expenses, including costs associated with medications, compression garments, wound care supplies, and healthcare visits, can impose a significant financial burden on patients and their families. Limited access to healthcare resources, insurance coverage, and financial assistance programs may further exacerbate financial strain and impact treatment adherence.
2. **Access to Care:** Geographic barriers, transportation

limitations, and healthcare disparities can hinder access to specialized care and comprehensive management for patients with chronic edema. Rural communities, underserved populations, and individuals with limited mobility or resources may face challenges in accessing lymphedema clinics, wound care centers, or multidisciplinary treatment programs.

Interventions and Supportive Strategies:

1. **Comprehensive Assessment:** A comprehensive assessment of patients with chronic edema should encompass physical, psychological, and social dimensions of well-being to identify underlying concerns, functional limitations, and support needs. Healthcare providers should utilize validated assessment tools, such as quality of life questionnaires or functional status scales, to evaluate the impact of edema on patient outcomes and guide treatment planning.
2. **Multidisciplinary Collaboration:** Multidisciplinary collaboration between healthcare providers, including physicians, nurses, physical therapists, occupational therapists, social workers, and psychologists, is essential for addressing the complex needs of patients with chronic edema. Integrated care teams can provide comprehensive assessment, personalized treatment planning, and coordinated support to optimize patient outcomes and enhance quality of life.
3. **Patient Education:** Patient education is key to empowering individuals with chronic edema to actively participate in their care, manage symptoms effectively, and make informed decisions about treatment options and self-care strategies. Education should encompass information about

edema management, skincare, compression therapy, physical activity, nutrition, and psychosocial support resources.

4. **Psychosocial Support:** Psychosocial support services, such as counseling, support groups, and peer mentoring, play a crucial role in addressing the emotional and social needs of patients with chronic edema. Providing a supportive environment, fostering peer connections, and offering coping strategies can help patients navigate the challenges of living with chronic edema and improve overall well-being.

5. **Functional Rehabilitation:** Functional rehabilitation programs focused on mobility training, strength conditioning, adaptive techniques, and assistive devices can help improve physical function and enhance independence in patients with chronic edema. Physical therapy interventions, such as manual lymphatic drainage (MLD), therapeutic exercise, and gait training, can optimize lymphatic drainage, reduce tissue swelling, and improve functional outcomes.

6. **Social Support Networks:** Building social support networks and community connections can help reduce feelings of isolation, loneliness, and social withdrawal in patients with chronic edema. Connecting patients with peer support groups, online forums, or community resources can foster a sense of belonging, provide emotional validation, and promote social engagement and participation.

Conclusion:

In conclusion, chronic edema exerts a profound impact on the quality of life and functional status of affected individuals, affecting physical health, emotional well-being, social relationships, and daily functioning. Understanding the multifaceted implications of chronic edema is essential for healthcare providers to implement supportive strategies, optimize treatment approaches, and improve overall patient outcomes. By addressing physical limitations, psychological distress, social implications, and practical challenges associated with chronic edema, healthcare providers can enhance patient well-being, promote functional independence, and improve overall quality of life for individuals living with this chronic condition.

Prognostic Factors and Long-Term Outcomes in Chronic Edema: Insights and Implications

Understanding prognostic factors and long-term outcomes is vital for effectively managing chronic edema, a condition characterized by persistent swelling due to fluid accumulation in the interstitial spaces of tissues. Prognostic factors help predict disease progression, treatment response, and overall prognosis, guiding healthcare providers in implementing personalized treatment plans and optimizing patient care. This exploration delves into the prognostic factors and long-term outcomes associated with chronic edema, encompassing clinical predictors, treatment considerations, and implications for patient management and quality of life.

Prognostic Factors:

1. **Underlying Etiology:** The underlying cause of chronic edema serves as a crucial prognostic factor, influencing disease progression, treatment response, and long-term outcomes. Etiologies such as lymphedema, venous insufficiency, heart failure, or renal dysfunction have distinct pathophysiological mechanisms and prognostic implications, requiring

tailored management approaches.

2. **Disease Severity:** The severity of chronic edema, characterized by the extent of tissue swelling, limb volume, and functional impairment, correlates with long-term outcomes and treatment response. Advanced stages of edema, marked by fibrosis, tissue changes, and recurrent infections, pose greater challenges in management and may have poorer prognoses.

3. **Comorbidities:** Comorbid conditions such as obesity, diabetes, hypertension, and peripheral vascular disease can exacerbate chronic edema, complicate treatment outcomes, and impact long-term prognosis. Comorbidities influence disease progression, treatment adherence, and risk of complications, necessitating comprehensive management strategies to address underlying health conditions.

4. **Lymphatic Dysfunction:** In cases of lymphedema or lymphatic insufficiency, the extent of lymphatic dysfunction, severity of lymphedema, and presence of associated complications such as cellulitis, lymphangitis, or lymphorrhea serve as prognostic indicators. Lymphatic imaging studies, lymphoscintigraphy, or lymphedema severity scores help assess lymphatic function and guide treatment planning.

5. **Venous Insufficiency:** Chronic venous insufficiency, characterized by venous reflux, venous hypertension, and venous stasis, is associated with complications such as venous ulcers, skin changes, and recurrent thrombosis, which impact long-term outcomes and prognosis. Duplex ultrasound, venous hemodynamic studies, and clinical staging systems aid in assessing venous insufficiency severity and guiding treatment decisions.

Long-Term Outcomes:

1. **Quality of Life:** Chronic edema significantly affects quality of life, resulting in physical limitations, emotional distress, social isolation, and impaired functional status. Long-term outcomes focus on improving quality of life through symptom management, functional rehabilitation, psychosocial support, and holistic care approaches that address physical, psychological, and social aspects of well-being.
2. **Functional Independence:** Long-term outcomes in chronic edema aim to enhance functional independence and optimize activities of daily living. Functional rehabilitation programs, including physical therapy, occupational therapy, and assistive devices, help improve mobility, strength, and manual dexterity, enabling patients to maintain independence and achieve their functional goals.
3. **Complication Prevention:** Long-term management of chronic edema focuses on preventing complications such as cellulitis, lymphangitis, venous ulcers, and impaired wound healing. Strategies for complication prevention include skincare, compression therapy, infection control, lymphedema education, and early intervention to address signs of infection or tissue breakdown.
4. **Treatment Adherence:** Long-term treatment outcomes in chronic edema depend on patient adherence to recommended interventions, including compression therapy, skincare, exercise, and self-management strategies. Patient education, counseling, and ongoing support are essential for promoting treatment adherence, empowering patients to actively participate in their care, and

optimizing long-term outcomes.
5. **Psychological Well-being:** Long-term management of chronic edema addresses the psychological impact of the condition, including anxiety, depression, body image concerns, and social isolation. Psychosocial support services, such as counseling, support groups, and peer mentoring, help address emotional needs, foster resilience, and improve overall psychological well-being.

Implications for Patient Management:

1. **Personalized Treatment Plans:** Prognostic factors in chronic edema inform the development of personalized treatment plans tailored to individual patient needs, disease severity, and prognostic indicators. Multidisciplinary care teams collaborate to assess prognostic factors, formulate treatment goals, and implement comprehensive management strategies that optimize patient outcomes and improve long-term prognosis.
2. **Regular Monitoring:** Long-term management of chronic edema involves regular monitoring of disease progression, treatment response, and complications to adjust treatment plans and optimize outcomes. Serial assessments, including clinical evaluations, imaging studies, lymphatic function tests, and quality of life assessments, help track changes over time and guide ongoing management decisions.
3. **Patient Education:** Patient education is essential for promoting self-management, treatment adherence, and lifestyle modifications that support long-term management of chronic edema. Patients receive education on skincare, compression therapy, exercise, nutrition, and psychosocial support resources to empower them to actively participate in their care and

optimize long-term outcomes.

4. **Shared Decision-Making:** Shared decision-making between healthcare providers and patients involves discussing treatment options, setting realistic goals, and addressing patient preferences and priorities. Collaborative care planning fosters patient engagement, enhances treatment adherence, and improves patient satisfaction with long-term management of chronic edema.

5. **Multidisciplinary Collaboration:** Multidisciplinary collaboration among healthcare providers, including physicians, nurses, therapists, and psychosocial support specialists, is essential for delivering comprehensive care to patients with chronic edema. Integrated care teams coordinate treatment plans, address complex needs, and optimize resources to improve patient outcomes and long-term prognosis.

Conclusion:

In conclusion, prognostic factors and long-term outcomes play a crucial role in the management of chronic edema, guiding treatment decisions, predicting disease progression, and optimizing patient care. Understanding the implications of prognostic factors and long-term outcomes helps healthcare providers develop personalized treatment plans, monitor disease progression, and address complications to improve quality of life and functional status in patients with chronic edema. By implementing comprehensive management strategies that address physical, psychological, and social aspects of well-being, healthcare providers can optimize long-term outcomes and enhance overall prognosis for individuals living with chronic edema.

CHAPTER 8: PREVENTION STRATEGIES AND PUBLIC HEALTH IMPLICATIONS

Primary Prevention of Chronic Edema: Lifestyle Modifications and Risk Factor Management

Preventing chronic edema requires a multifaceted approach that addresses underlying risk factors, promotes healthy lifestyle habits, and implements preventive measures to reduce the incidence and progression of fluid accumulation in the interstitial spaces of tissues. Primary prevention strategies focus on lifestyle modifications, risk factor management, and health promotion initiatives aimed at minimizing modifiable risk factors and optimizing overall health and well-being. This exploration delves into primary prevention of chronic edema, encompassing lifestyle modifications, risk factor identification, and practical interventions to promote fluid balance, vascular health, and lymphatic function, providing insights into effective strategies for reducing the burden of chronic edema on individuals and healthcare systems.

Lifestyle Modifications:

1. **Maintaining a Healthy Weight:** Obesity is a significant risk factor for chronic edema, as excess adipose tissue can exert pressure on blood vessels and impair lymphatic drainage, leading to fluid retention and tissue swelling. Encouraging individuals to maintain a healthy weight through balanced nutrition, regular physical activity, and portion control can help reduce the risk of developing obesity-related edema.
2. **Regular Exercise:** Physical activity plays a crucial role in promoting vascular health, improving lymphatic function, and reducing the risk of chronic edema. Engaging in regular exercise, including aerobic activities, strength training, and flexibility exercises, helps enhance circulation, promote lymphatic drainage, and maintain muscle tone, contributing to overall fluid balance and tissue health.
3. **Healthy Diet:** A balanced diet rich in fruits, vegetables, whole grains, lean proteins, and healthy fats supports vascular health, reduces inflammation, and promotes optimal fluid balance. Encouraging individuals to consume a diet low in sodium, processed foods, and saturated fats can help minimize fluid retention and mitigate the risk of developing edema-related conditions such as hypertension and heart failure.
4. **Hydration Management:** Adequate hydration is essential for maintaining fluid balance and supporting lymphatic function. Encouraging individuals to drink plenty of water throughout the day and limit consumption of dehydrating beverages such as caffeine and alcohol helps prevent dehydration, optimize lymphatic drainage, and reduce the risk of

fluid accumulation in tissues.

5. **Compression Garments:** Wearing compression garments or stockings can help prevent fluid buildup in the lower extremities, improve venous return, and reduce the risk of venous insufficiency-related edema. Recommending compression therapy for individuals at risk of developing edema, such as those with a history of venous thrombosis or prolonged standing, can help promote vascular health and prevent fluid retention.

Risk Factor Management:

1. **Venous Insufficiency:** Managing risk factors for venous insufficiency, such as prolonged sitting or standing, obesity, pregnancy, and hormonal contraceptives, is essential for preventing venous-related edema. Encouraging individuals to elevate their legs, wear compression stockings, and engage in regular physical activity can help improve venous circulation and reduce the risk of venous insufficiency-related complications.

2. **Lymphatic Dysfunction:** Identifying and managing risk factors for lymphatic dysfunction, such as trauma, surgery, infection, or genetic predisposition, is critical for preventing lymphedema and related complications. Educating individuals about early signs of lymphatic impairment, promoting skincare, and encouraging regular exercise and manual lymphatic drainage techniques can help support lymphatic function and reduce the risk of lymphedema development.

3. **Heart Failure:** Managing risk factors for heart failure, including hypertension, coronary artery disease, diabetes, and obesity, is essential for preventing fluid overload and edema formation. Encouraging

individuals to monitor their blood pressure, adhere to prescribed medications, follow a heart-healthy diet, and engage in regular exercise can help optimize cardiovascular health and reduce the risk of heart failure-related edema.

4. **Renal Dysfunction:** Preventing renal dysfunction and chronic kidney disease through lifestyle modifications, including maintaining a healthy weight, managing blood pressure, and avoiding nephrotoxic medications, is crucial for preventing fluid retention and edema formation. Encouraging individuals to stay hydrated, monitor their kidney function, and undergo regular screening for kidney disease risk factors can help preserve renal function and mitigate the risk of renal-related edema.

5. **Inflammatory Disorders:** Managing inflammatory disorders such as rheumatoid arthritis, lupus, or inflammatory bowel disease through medication management, lifestyle modifications, and regular monitoring is essential for preventing inflammation-related edema. Collaborating with rheumatologists, immunologists, or gastroenterologists to optimize disease control and minimize inflammatory flares can help reduce the risk of chronic edema in individuals with autoimmune or inflammatory conditions.

Practical Interventions:

1. **Patient Education:** Educating individuals about the importance of preventive measures, early symptom recognition, and self-care strategies is essential for empowering them to take proactive steps in managing their health and reducing the risk of chronic edema. Providing information about lifestyle modifications, risk factor management, and early intervention for fluid retention symptoms can help promote patient

engagement and adherence to preventive measures.

2. **Community Outreach:** Community-based health promotion initiatives, including health fairs, educational workshops, and outreach programs, play a vital role in raising awareness about chronic edema, risk factors, and preventive strategies. Collaborating with community organizations, schools, workplaces, and local health departments to disseminate information, promote healthy behaviors, and encourage early intervention can help reach individuals at risk of developing edema-related conditions.

3. **Occupational Health Programs:** Implementing occupational health programs that address ergonomic factors, workplace hazards, and occupational risks for edema development can help prevent work-related injuries and promote vascular health. Providing education, ergonomic assessments, and workplace modifications tailored to specific job tasks and occupational hazards can help reduce the risk of occupational-related edema in high-risk populations.

4. **Home-Based Interventions:** Offering home-based interventions such as telehealth consultations, home exercise programs, and self-care resources can help individuals implement preventive measures and manage chronic edema from the comfort of their homes. Telehealth platforms, mobile health apps, and remote monitoring devices facilitate virtual consultations, self-management education, and adherence support, improving access to care and promoting patient engagement in preventive interventions.

Conclusion:

In conclusion, primary prevention of chronic edema requires

a proactive approach that addresses modifiable risk factors, promotes healthy lifestyle habits, and implements practical interventions to reduce the incidence and progression of fluid accumulation in tissues. Lifestyle modifications, risk factor management, and health promotion initiatives play a crucial role in preventing chronic edema-related conditions such as venous insufficiency, lymphedema, heart failure, renal dysfunction, and inflammatory disorders. By empowering individuals with knowledge, resources, and support to adopt healthy behaviors, manage underlying risk factors, and recognize early signs of fluid retention, healthcare providers can promote vascular health, optimize lymphatic function, and reduce the burden of chronic edema on individuals and society.

Secondary Prevention: Early Detection and Management of Precursor Conditions to Prevent Chronic Edema

Secondary prevention strategies focus on the early detection and management of precursor conditions that predispose individuals to develop chronic edema. By identifying and addressing risk factors, underlying diseases, and early signs of fluid retention, healthcare providers can intervene at an early stage to prevent the progression to chronic edema and its associated complications. This exploration delves into secondary prevention of chronic edema, encompassing screening protocols, diagnostic strategies, and targeted interventions aimed at identifying and managing precursor conditions, providing insights into effective strategies for reducing the burden of chronic edema on individuals and healthcare systems.

Early Detection Strategies:

1. **Comprehensive Screening:** Implementing comprehensive screening protocols to identify individuals at risk of developing chronic edema is essential for secondary prevention efforts. Screening may include medical history review, assessment of risk factors (e.g., obesity, venous insufficiency, lymphatic dysfunction), physical examination, and diagnostic tests such as ultrasound, lymphoscintigraphy, or laboratory tests to evaluate vascular and lymphatic function.
2. **Risk Factor Assessment:** Assessing modifiable risk factors such as obesity, sedentary lifestyle, occupational hazards, and comorbid conditions is crucial for identifying individuals at increased risk of developing chronic edema. Risk factor assessment may involve standardized questionnaires, physical assessment tools, and collaboration with multidisciplinary healthcare providers to evaluate vascular, lymphatic, and metabolic health.
3. **Symptom Recognition:** Educating individuals about early signs and symptoms of fluid retention, such as swelling, heaviness, discomfort, or skin changes, empowers them to recognize warning signs and seek timely medical evaluation. Promoting awareness about edema-related symptoms through public health campaigns, patient education materials, and community outreach initiatives facilitates early detection and intervention.

Diagnostic Strategies:

1. **Clinical Evaluation:** A thorough clinical evaluation, including medical history review, physical examination, and assessment of edema-related symptoms, is essential for diagnosing precursor conditions and identifying individuals at risk of

developing chronic edema. Clinical signs such as pitting edema, skin changes, venous varicosities, or lymphatic congestion provide valuable diagnostic clues and guide further evaluation.
2. **Imaging Studies:** Diagnostic imaging modalities such as ultrasound, Doppler studies, magnetic resonance imaging (MRI), or computed tomography (CT) scans play a crucial role in evaluating vascular and lymphatic function, identifying structural abnormalities, and confirming the presence of precursor conditions such as venous insufficiency, lymphatic obstruction, or organ dysfunction.
3. **Lymphatic Function Tests:** Specialized tests such as lymphoscintigraphy, lymphangiography, or indocyanine green (ICG) lymphography are valuable tools for assessing lymphatic function, detecting lymphatic abnormalities, and diagnosing lymphatic disorders such as lymphedema or lymphatic leakage. Lymphatic function tests provide objective data on lymphatic drainage capacity, transit times, and lymphatic architecture, guiding treatment decisions and monitoring disease progression.

Targeted Interventions:

1. **Early Treatment Initiatives:** Early intervention in precursor conditions such as venous insufficiency, lymphatic dysfunction, heart failure, renal impairment, or inflammatory disorders is essential for preventing the progression to chronic edema. Targeted interventions may include lifestyle modifications, pharmacological therapy, compression therapy, physical therapy, or surgical procedures tailored to the underlying etiology and disease severity.
2. **Pharmacological Management:** Pharmacological interventions such as diuretics, vasodilators, anti-

inflammatory agents, or medications targeting underlying comorbidities (e.g., hypertension, diabetes, autoimmune disorders) play a crucial role in managing precursor conditions and preventing fluid retention. Pharmacotherapy aims to improve vascular function, reduce inflammation, optimize fluid balance, and mitigate the risk of developing chronic edema-related complications.

3. **Compression Therapy:** Compression therapy, including compression stockings, bandages, or pneumatic compression devices, is a cornerstone of treatment for precursor conditions such as venous insufficiency, lymphatic dysfunction, or post-surgical edema. Compression garments exert external pressure on tissues, enhance venous return, promote lymphatic drainage, and reduce tissue swelling, preventing the progression to chronic edema and improving overall vascular health.

4. **Physical Rehabilitation:** Physical rehabilitation programs, including exercise therapy, manual lymphatic drainage (MLD), therapeutic exercises, and rehabilitation techniques, help improve vascular function, promote lymphatic drainage, and prevent the development of chronic edema. Physical therapists collaborate with patients to develop personalized exercise regimens, optimize mobility, and enhance functional status, reducing the risk of fluid retention and improving overall health outcomes.

Integrated Care Approach:

1. **Multidisciplinary Collaboration:** Multidisciplinary collaboration among healthcare providers, including primary care physicians, specialists (e.g., vascular surgeons, cardiologists, nephrologists, rheumatologists), nurses, physical therapists, and

occupational therapists, is essential for implementing integrated care approaches to secondary prevention of chronic edema. Coordinated care teams collaborate to assess risk factors, diagnose precursor conditions, and implement targeted interventions tailored to individual patient needs and disease complexity.

2. **Patient-Centered Care:** Patient-centered care models prioritize individualized treatment plans, shared decision-making, and patient engagement in managing precursor conditions and preventing chronic edema. Empowering patients through education, self-management strategies, and ongoing support facilitates active participation in their care, promotes treatment adherence, and improves long-term health outcomes.

3. **Continuity of Care:** Ensuring continuity of care through regular follow-up visits, monitoring disease progression, and adjusting treatment plans as needed is essential for maintaining optimal health outcomes and preventing the recurrence of fluid retention. Coordinated care transitions, communication between healthcare providers, and patient education on self-monitoring techniques promote seamless care delivery and empower individuals to take charge of their health.

Conclusion:

In conclusion, secondary prevention of chronic edema focuses on early detection and management of precursor conditions to prevent the progression to fluid retention and associated complications. Comprehensive screening, risk factor assessment, symptom recognition, and diagnostic evaluation facilitate early intervention, targeted treatment strategies, and optimal health outcomes. By implementing integrated care approaches, promoting patient-centered care, and ensuring continuity of care, healthcare providers can effectively identify individuals at risk of developing chronic edema, intervene at an early stage, and prevent the burden of this chronic condition on individuals and healthcare systems.

Tertiary Prevention: Rehabilitation and Long-Term Care for Chronic Edema

Tertiary prevention strategies aim to minimize the impact of chronic edema on individuals' quality of life, functional status, and overall well-being through rehabilitation and long-term care interventions. By addressing residual impairments, managing complications, and optimizing functional outcomes, tertiary prevention efforts support individuals with chronic edema in achieving maximal independence, participation, and quality of life. This exploration delves into tertiary prevention of chronic edema, encompassing rehabilitation approaches, wound care management, psychosocial support, and palliative care strategies, providing insights into comprehensive interventions for optimizing long-term outcomes and promoting holistic well-being.

Rehabilitation Approaches:

1. **Physical Therapy:** Physical therapy plays a central role in tertiary prevention of chronic edema by focusing on improving mobility, strength, flexibility, and functional independence. Physical therapists design personalized exercise programs, manual lymphatic drainage techniques, and therapeutic interventions to promote lymphatic drainage, reduce tissue swelling, and enhance overall physical function.

2. **Occupational Therapy:** Occupational therapists assist individuals with chronic edema in regaining independence in activities of daily living (ADLs) and instrumental activities of daily living (IADLs) through adaptive techniques, assistive devices, and environmental modifications. Occupational therapy interventions aim to optimize self-care skills, promote energy conservation, and facilitate participation in meaningful activities despite functional limitations.
3. **Speech Therapy:** Speech therapy may be indicated for individuals with chronic edema-related complications such as dysphagia (swallowing difficulties) or dysphonia (voice disorders) secondary to head and neck edema. Speech therapists assess swallowing function, recommend dietary modifications, and provide exercises to improve swallowing safety and vocal quality, enhancing communication and nutritional status.
4. **Rehabilitation Engineering:** Rehabilitation engineers design custom orthoses, prostheses, assistive devices, and adaptive equipment to address functional limitations and support individuals with chronic edema in performing daily activities. Assistive technology solutions such as compression garments, mobility aids, and ergonomic tools promote independence, safety, and quality of life in individuals with chronic edema-related impairments.

Wound Care Management:

1. **Comprehensive Wound Assessment:** Tertiary prevention of chronic edema involves comprehensive wound assessment to identify underlying etiology, assess wound characteristics, and determine appropriate wound care interventions. Healthcare providers conduct thorough evaluations of wound

size, depth, drainage, tissue perfusion, and surrounding skin condition to guide treatment decisions and monitor healing progress.

2. **Advanced Wound Care Interventions:** Advanced wound care interventions such as debridement, wound irrigation, dressings, and topical agents are tailored to the specific needs of individuals with chronic edema-related wounds. Moisture-retentive dressings, antimicrobial dressings, and biological agents promote optimal wound healing, prevent infection, and create a conducive environment for tissue regeneration.

3. **Compression Therapy:** Compression therapy is a cornerstone of wound care management in individuals with chronic edema, as it helps reduce tissue swelling, improve venous return, and promote wound healing. Graduated compression garments, multi-layer compression bandages, or intermittent pneumatic compression devices are utilized to apply controlled pressure to the affected area, facilitating edema reduction and wound closure.

4. **Negative Pressure Wound Therapy (NPWT):** NPWT may be indicated for individuals with chronic edema-related wounds that are slow to heal or have complex etiologies. NPWT promotes wound healing by creating a negative pressure environment, removing excess fluid, improving tissue perfusion, and stimulating granulation tissue formation, leading to expedited wound closure and improved outcomes.

Psychosocial Support:

1. **Counseling and Psychotherapy:** Psychosocial support services, including counseling, psychotherapy, and support groups, play a crucial role in addressing the emotional and psychological impact of chronic

edema on individuals and their families. Mental health professionals provide coping strategies, emotional support, and stress management techniques to help individuals navigate the challenges of living with chronic edema and promote psychological resilience.

2. **Peer Support Networks:** Peer support networks, online forums, and community-based organizations provide opportunities for individuals with chronic edema to connect with others facing similar challenges, share experiences, and exchange practical tips for self-management. Peer mentoring programs offer peer-to-peer support, encouragement, and validation, fostering a sense of belonging and empowerment among individuals with chronic edema.

3. **Education and Self-Management:** Education programs and self-management interventions empower individuals with chronic edema to actively participate in their care, monitor symptoms, and implement preventive strategies. Educational resources, self-care guides, and online tools facilitate access to information, promote self-advocacy, and enhance individuals' ability to manage their condition effectively.

Palliative Care Strategies:

1. **Symptom Management:** Palliative care focuses on relieving symptoms, improving comfort, and enhancing quality of life in individuals with chronic edema, particularly those with advanced or incurable conditions. Symptom management interventions address pain, discomfort, fatigue, anxiety, and other distressing symptoms associated with chronic edema-related complications, optimizing comfort and well-being.

2. **End-of-Life Care Planning:** Palliative care teams collaborate with individuals with chronic edema and their families to develop comprehensive end-of-life care plans that align with their values, preferences, and goals of care. Advance care planning discussions, goals-of-care conversations, and support for decision-making facilitate informed choices, ensure dignity, and promote a peaceful end-of-life experience.
3. **Family Support:** Palliative care extends support to families and caregivers of individuals with chronic edema, addressing their emotional, practical, and spiritual needs throughout the caregiving journey. Counseling, respite care services, bereavement support, and caregiver education programs help alleviate caregiver burden, foster resilience, and promote well-being in family members and loved ones.

Conclusion:

In conclusion, tertiary prevention of chronic edema focuses on rehabilitation and long-term care interventions aimed at optimizing functional outcomes, managing complications, and enhancing quality of life in affected individuals. Comprehensive rehabilitation approaches, wound care management strategies, psychosocial support services, and palliative care interventions address the multidimensional needs of individuals with chronic edema, promoting holistic well-being and maximizing independence, participation, and dignity throughout the care continuum. By implementing integrated care models, fostering interdisciplinary collaboration, and prioritizing patient-centered approaches, healthcare providers can effectively support individuals with chronic edema in achieving optimal health outcomes and enhancing overall quality of life.

Public Health Initiatives and Educational Campaigns for Chronic Edema

Public health initiatives and educational campaigns play a pivotal role in raising awareness, promoting early detection, and implementing preventive strategies for chronic edema. By engaging communities, healthcare professionals, policymakers, and stakeholders, these initiatives aim to reduce the burden of chronic edema, improve health outcomes, and enhance quality of life for affected individuals. This exploration delves into public health initiatives and educational campaigns for chronic edema, encompassing awareness-raising efforts, screening programs, health promotion activities, and advocacy initiatives, providing insights into effective strategies for addressing this complex health issue at the population level.

Awareness-Raising Efforts:

1. **Public Awareness Campaigns:** Public awareness campaigns utilize various media channels, including television, radio, print media, social media, and online platforms, to disseminate information about chronic edema, its risk factors, early signs, and preventive measures. These campaigns aim to educate the general public, raise awareness about the importance of early detection, and promote timely intervention to prevent the progression of chronic edema-related conditions.
2. **Community Outreach Events:** Community outreach events such as health fairs, wellness workshops, and educational seminars provide opportunities for direct engagement with individuals, families, and communities. These events offer interactive sessions,

health screenings, and informational booths focused on chronic edema awareness, risk factor identification, and lifestyle modifications to promote vascular health and lymphatic function.

3. **Celebrity Endorsements and Public Figures:** Collaborating with celebrities, public figures, and influential personalities can amplify the reach and impact of chronic edema awareness campaigns. Celebrity endorsements, public testimonials, and personal stories raise visibility, generate media interest, and mobilize public support for preventive measures, encouraging individuals to prioritize their vascular and lymphatic health.

Screening Programs:

1. **Community-Based Screening Clinics:** Community-based screening clinics provide accessible, convenient, and cost-effective opportunities for individuals to undergo screening tests for chronic edema-related risk factors and early signs. These clinics may offer free or subsidized screenings for venous insufficiency, lymphatic dysfunction, obesity, and other predisposing factors, enabling early detection and intervention.

2. **School and Workplace Health Programs:** School and workplace health programs incorporate chronic edema screening components into existing health promotion initiatives, wellness programs, and employee health benefits. Screening activities may include health risk assessments, body composition analyses, and vascular health screenings to identify individuals at risk and promote preventive measures through education and outreach efforts.

3. **Mobile Health (mHealth) Applications:** Mobile health applications and digital health platforms

offer innovative tools for self-assessment, symptom tracking, and health monitoring related to chronic edema. These apps provide educational resources, self-care tips, and personalized risk assessments, empowering users to take proactive steps in managing their vascular and lymphatic health and seek timely medical attention when needed.

Health Promotion Activities:

1. **Educational Workshops and Webinars:** Educational workshops, webinars, and online learning modules provide in-depth information about chronic edema, its pathophysiology, risk factors, and management strategies. These educational sessions are conducted by healthcare professionals, patient advocacy groups, and community organizations, offering interactive discussions, Q&A sessions, and practical tips for prevention and self-management.
2. **Patient Education Materials:** Patient education materials, including brochures, pamphlets, fact sheets, and multimedia resources, are valuable tools for disseminating information about chronic edema to individuals, families, and caregivers. These materials address common questions, dispel myths, and provide guidance on lifestyle modifications, self-care practices, and when to seek medical attention for edema-related concerns.
3. **Online Support Communities:** Online support communities, forums, and social media groups bring together individuals with chronic edema, caregivers, and healthcare professionals to share experiences, exchange information, and provide peer support. These virtual communities offer a platform for emotional support, practical advice, and encouragement, fostering a sense of belonging and

empowerment among individuals living with chronic edema.

Advocacy Initiatives:

1. **Policy Advocacy and Legislative Efforts:** Advocacy organizations and patient advocacy groups advocate for policies and legislation that support individuals with chronic edema, improve access to care, and advance research and innovation in vascular and lymphatic health. Advocacy efforts may focus on insurance coverage for compression therapy, funding for research initiatives, and inclusion of lymphedema management in healthcare policies.
2. **Health Equity and Access Campaigns:** Health equity and access campaigns address disparities in access to care and resources for individuals with chronic edema, particularly underserved and marginalized populations. These campaigns advocate for equitable access to preventive services, diagnostic testing, treatment options, and supportive care services, ensuring that all individuals have the opportunity to manage their condition effectively and improve their health outcomes.
3. **Professional Training and Continuing Education:** Advocacy organizations collaborate with healthcare professional associations, academic institutions, and training programs to enhance professional education and competency in chronic edema management. Continuing education initiatives, workshops, and certification programs provide healthcare providers with up-to-date knowledge, skills, and best practices for diagnosing, treating, and supporting individuals with chronic edema across diverse healthcare settings.

Conclusion:

In conclusion, public health initiatives and educational campaigns play a critical role in raising awareness, promoting early detection, and implementing preventive strategies for chronic edema. By engaging communities, healthcare professionals, policymakers, and stakeholders, these initiatives foster a culture of vascular and lymphatic health, empower individuals to take proactive steps in managing their condition, and promote equity in access to care and resources. Through collaborative efforts, advocacy initiatives, and innovative approaches to health promotion, we can reduce the burden of chronic edema, improve health outcomes, and enhance quality of life for individuals living with this chronic condition.

CHAPTER 9: EMERGING RESEARCH AND FUTURE DIRECTIONS

Advances in Understanding Edema Pathophysiology

Over the past decades, significant advances have been made in our understanding of the pathophysiology of edema, shedding light on the complex interplay of cellular, molecular, and systemic factors underlying fluid accumulation in tissues. These advancements have provided valuable insights into the mechanisms driving edema formation, facilitating the development of targeted therapeutic approaches and preventive strategies. This exploration delves into recent advances in understanding edema pathophysiology, encompassing cellular mechanisms, molecular pathways, and systemic factors contributing to fluid imbalance, providing insights into the intricate processes involved in edema development and progression.

1. Cellular Mechanisms of Edema:

Recent research has elucidated the cellular mechanisms involved in edema formation, highlighting the role of endothelial cells, epithelial cells, and inflammatory mediators in modulating vascular permeability and fluid movement across tissue compartments. Endothelial dysfunction, characterized by increased vascular permeability and impaired barrier function, disrupts the balance between fluid filtration and reabsorption, leading to extravasation of plasma proteins and fluid accumulation in interstitial spaces.

Endothelial activation, triggered by inflammatory cytokines, vasoactive substances, and oxidative stress, promotes the expression of adhesion molecules, cytokines, and chemokines, facilitating leukocyte recruitment, capillary leakage, and tissue inflammation. Epithelial dysfunction in organs such as the lungs, kidneys, and gastrointestinal tract further exacerbates fluid retention by impairing sodium transport, water reabsorption, and electrolyte balance, contributing to organ-specific edema formation.

Recent studies have also highlighted the role of lymphatic dysfunction in edema pathophysiology, emphasizing the importance of lymphatic vessels in maintaining fluid homeostasis, immune surveillance, and tissue drainage. Lymphatic obstruction, impaired lymphatic contractility, or lymphatic vessel insufficiency compromise lymphatic drainage capacity, resulting in lymphedema, tissue congestion, and impaired immune function.

2. Molecular Pathways Driving Edema Formation:

Advances in molecular biology and biochemistry have identified key signaling pathways and molecular mediators implicated in edema pathogenesis, providing potential targets for pharmacological intervention and therapeutic modulation. Vascular endothelial growth factor (VEGF), a potent angiogenic factor and permeability enhancer, plays a central role in promoting vascular leakage, endothelial dysfunction, and edema formation in various pathological conditions.

Inflammatory cytokines such as tumor necrosis factor-alpha (TNF-α), interleukin-1 (IL-1), and interleukin-6 (IL-6) orchestrate a pro-inflammatory cascade, activating endothelial cells, recruiting immune cells, and promoting vasodilation and vascular permeability. Matrix metalloproteinases (MMPs), enzymes involved in extracellular matrix remodeling, degrade vascular basement membranes, disrupt cell-cell junctions, and facilitate leukocyte extravasation, exacerbating tissue injury and edema progression.

Recent studies have also implicated the renin-angiotensin-aldosterone system (RAAS) in edema pathophysiology, highlighting the role of angiotensin II, aldosterone, and endothelin-1 in promoting vasoconstriction, sodium retention, and fluid accumulation. Dysregulation of RAAS signaling, observed in conditions such as heart failure, renal dysfunction, and hypertension, contributes to volume overload, venous congestion, and edema formation, underscoring the importance of targeting RAAS components in edema management.

3. Systemic Factors Influencing Edema Development:

Advances in systems biology and integrative physiology have elucidated the systemic factors influencing edema development and progression, including fluid balance regulation, neurohormonal control, and microcirculatory dysfunction. Dysregulation of fluid balance mechanisms, such as altered hydrostatic pressure, oncotic pressure, and lymphatic drainage, disrupts the equilibrium between fluid filtration and absorption, predisposing individuals to edema formation.

Neurohormonal factors, including sympathetic nervous system activation, antidiuretic hormone (ADH) release, and atrial natriuretic peptide (ANP) secretion, modulate renal sodium handling, water reabsorption, and vascular tone, influencing intravascular volume status and extracellular fluid distribution. Dysfunctional neurohormonal signaling, observed in conditions such as heart failure, cirrhosis, and renal impairment, impairs fluid homeostasis, exacerbating fluid retention and edema progression.

Microcirculatory dysfunction, characterized by impaired capillary perfusion, tissue hypoxia, and endothelial dysfunction, contributes to edema formation by disrupting microvascular integrity, impairing oxygen delivery, and promoting inflammatory cell infiltration. Recent advancements in microvascular imaging techniques, such as intravital microscopy and laser Doppler flowmetry, have provided valuable insights into microcirculatory alterations underlying edema pathophysiology, facilitating targeted interventions to improve tissue perfusion and oxygenation.

Conclusion:

In conclusion, recent advances in understanding edema pathophysiology have unraveled the intricate cellular mechanisms, molecular pathways, and systemic factors driving fluid imbalance and tissue congestion. By elucidating the role of endothelial dysfunction, inflammatory mediators, lymphatic impairment, molecular signaling pathways, and systemic dysregulation in edema development, these advancements have paved the way for innovative therapeutic approaches and preventive strategies aimed at mitigating edema burden and improving clinical outcomes. Continued research efforts aimed at unraveling the complexities of edema pathophysiology hold promise for the development of personalized interventions and precision medicine approaches tailored to the individual needs of patients with edema-related conditions.

Novel Therapeutic Targets and Treatment Modalities for Edema

The quest for more effective therapies to manage edema has led to the exploration of novel therapeutic targets and treatment modalities. Recent advancements in pharmacology, biotechnology, and medical devices have expanded the armamentarium of treatment options, offering promising avenues for addressing the underlying pathophysiology of edema and improving patient outcomes. This exploration delves into emerging therapeutic targets and innovative treatment modalities for edema, encompassing pharmacological agents, biologics, medical devices, and regenerative medicine approaches, providing insights into the evolving landscape of edema management.

1. Pharmacological Agents:

Recent research has identified novel pharmacological targets and therapeutic agents for edema management, offering potential avenues for modulating vascular permeability, lymphatic function, and fluid balance regulation. These pharmacological agents target key pathways involved in edema pathophysiology, including endothelial dysfunction, inflammation, and neurohormonal dysregulation, providing opportunities for personalized treatment approaches tailored to the underlying etiology of edema.

Endothelial Barrier Modulators: Novel pharmacological agents targeting endothelial barrier function, such as angiopoietin-1 (Ang-1) mimetics, sphingosine-1-phosphate (S1P) receptor agonists, and vascular endothelial growth factor (VEGF) inhibitors, hold promise for stabilizing vascular integrity, reducing vascular leakage, and mitigating edema formation in various pathological conditions.

Anti-inflammatory Agents: Anti-inflammatory agents targeting cytokines, chemokines, and inflammatory mediators implicated in edema pathogenesis, including interleukin-1 (IL-1) inhibitors, tumor necrosis factor-alpha (TNF-α) antagonists, and nuclear factor kappa B (NF-κB) inhibitors, offer potential therapeutic benefits in mitigating endothelial activation, leukocyte recruitment, and tissue inflammation associated with edema.

Neurohormonal Modulators: Pharmacological agents targeting neurohormonal pathways involved in fluid balance regulation, such as vasopressin receptor antagonists, aldosterone antagonists, and renin inhibitors, provide opportunities for optimizing renal sodium excretion, water balance, and vascular tone, thereby reducing volume overload and edema progression in conditions such as heart failure and renal impairment.

2. Biologics and Targeted Therapies:

Biologics and targeted therapies represent a promising approach for edema management, leveraging the specificity and potency of biologically active molecules to modulate key molecular pathways implicated in edema pathophysiology. These innovative therapies target specific cellular receptors, signaling pathways, and molecular mediators involved in vascular permeability, lymphatic function, and inflammatory responses, offering targeted interventions with potential for improved efficacy and safety profiles.

Monoclonal Antibodies: Monoclonal antibodies targeting pro-inflammatory cytokines, growth factors, and cell surface receptors involved in edema pathogenesis, such as VEGF, TNF-α, and endothelin-1 (ET-1), offer targeted blockade of pathological pathways, reducing vascular leakage, inflammation, and tissue injury associated with edema.

Lymphangiogenic Factors: Lymphangiogenic factors, including vascular endothelial growth factor-C (VEGF-C) and lymphatic vessel endothelial hyaluronan receptor-1 (LYVE-1) agonists, promote lymphatic vessel growth, lymphatic drainage, and tissue fluid clearance, offering potential therapeutic benefits in conditions characterized by lymphatic dysfunction and lymphedema.

Gene Therapy: Gene therapy approaches targeting genes involved in lymphatic development, lymphatic function, or vascular integrity hold promise for restoring lymphatic drainage capacity, enhancing tissue fluid clearance, and mitigating edema progression. Gene transfer vectors, such as viral vectors or nanoparticle-based delivery systems, enable targeted gene delivery to specific tissues or cell types, offering potential for personalized treatment approaches tailored to the underlying genetic defects in lymphatic disorders.

3. Medical Devices and Interventional Therapies:

Advancements in medical devices and interventional therapies have expanded treatment options for edema management, offering minimally invasive approaches for fluid removal, lymphatic drainage enhancement, and tissue decompression. These innovative modalities leverage technology-driven solutions to address the mechanical, physiological, and anatomical aspects of edema pathophysiology, providing targeted interventions with potential for improved efficacy and patient compliance.

Compression Therapy Devices: Advanced compression therapy devices, including pneumatic compression pumps, intermittent compression sleeves, and multilayer compression bandages, deliver controlled pressure to the affected limbs, promoting venous return, lymphatic drainage, and tissue decongestion in individuals with venous insufficiency, lymphedema, or post-surgical edema.

Lymphatic Interventional Procedures: Interventional procedures targeting the lymphatic system, such as lymphaticovenous anastomosis (LVA), lymphatic embolization, and lymphatic vessel transplantation, offer minimally invasive approaches for enhancing lymphatic drainage, bypassing obstructed lymphatic channels, and restoring tissue fluid balance in patients with lymphatic disorders and lymphedema.

Surgical Decompression Techniques: Surgical decompression techniques, such as fasciotomy, aponeurotomy, and subcutaneous tissue release, provide definitive treatment options for severe cases of edema-related compartment syndrome, chronic venous insufficiency, or lymphedema, relieving tissue pressure, improving microcirculation, and preventing tissue ischemia and necrosis.

Conclusion:

In conclusion, novel therapeutic targets and treatment modalities hold promise for advancing the management of edema, offering targeted interventions tailored to the underlying pathophysiology of fluid imbalance and tissue congestion. Pharmacological agents, biologics, medical devices, and interventional therapies provide innovative approaches for modulating vascular permeability, lymphatic function, and fluid balance regulation, offering opportunities for personalized treatment strategies and improved clinical outcomes in individuals with edema-related conditions. Continued research efforts and clinical trials are needed to further elucidate the efficacy, safety, and long-term benefits of these emerging therapies, paving the way for enhanced edema management and improved quality of life for affected individuals.

CHAPTER 10: INTEGRATIVE AND HOLISTIC PERSPECTIVES

Role of Nutrition and Nutraceuticals in Edema Management

Nutrition plays a crucial role in the management of edema, influencing fluid balance, tissue integrity, and inflammatory processes. By adopting a balanced diet rich in nutrients and incorporating specific nutraceuticals, individuals with edema can support lymphatic function, reduce inflammation, and promote tissue healing, complementing conventional treatment approaches. This exploration delves into the role of nutrition and nutraceuticals in edema management, encompassing dietary strategies, micronutrient supplementation, and herbal remedies, providing insights into holistic approaches to optimize fluid balance and support overall health.

1. Dietary Strategies for Edema Management:

A well-balanced diet is essential for maintaining fluid balance, supporting lymphatic function, and reducing inflammation, key components of edema management. Dietary strategies focus on optimizing nutrient intake, minimizing sodium consumption, and incorporating foods with anti-inflammatory and diuretic properties, promoting overall health and well-being.

Hydration: Adequate hydration is essential for maintaining fluid balance and supporting lymphatic drainage. Individuals with edema should aim to consume sufficient fluids, primarily water, throughout the day to prevent dehydration and promote urine output. Herbal teas, coconut water, and electrolyte-rich beverages can also contribute to hydration while providing additional health benefits.

Sodium Restriction: Excessive sodium intake contributes to fluid retention and exacerbates edema by increasing extracellular fluid volume and impairing renal sodium excretion. Dietary sodium restriction is recommended for individuals with edema, aiming to limit sodium intake to less than 2,300 milligrams per day (equivalent to about one teaspoon of salt) and preferably lower for those with hypertension or heart failure.

Potassium-Rich Foods: Potassium-rich foods, such as bananas, oranges, spinach, and sweet potatoes, help counteract the sodium-induced fluid retention by promoting diuresis and urinary sodium excretion. Including potassium-rich foods in the diet can help restore electrolyte balance and support cardiovascular health, reducing the risk of edema-related complications.

Anti-inflammatory Foods: Incorporating anti-inflammatory foods into the diet, such as fatty fish (salmon, mackerel), nuts, seeds, fruits (berries, cherries), and vegetables (leafy greens, broccoli), helps mitigate inflammation and oxidative stress, common contributors to edema formation. These foods provide essential nutrients, antioxidants, and omega-3 fatty acids, promoting tissue healing and reducing inflammatory cytokine production.

Protein Adequacy: Adequate protein intake is essential for maintaining tissue integrity, supporting wound healing, and preserving lean muscle mass in individuals with edema. Including lean protein sources, such as poultry, fish, legumes, and tofu, in the diet ensures sufficient amino acid supply for tissue repair and regeneration, promoting overall health and recovery.

2. Micronutrient Supplementation:

Micronutrient deficiencies can exacerbate edema and impair immune function, highlighting the importance of micronutrient supplementation in individuals with nutritional deficiencies or specific medical conditions. Targeted supplementation with vitamins, minerals, and antioxidants can help address underlying nutrient deficiencies, support lymphatic function, and enhance tissue repair processes, contributing to edema management and overall health.

Vitamin C: Vitamin C plays a critical role in collagen synthesis, immune function, and antioxidant defense mechanisms, essential for maintaining vascular integrity and supporting tissue healing in individuals with edema. Supplementation with vitamin C can help reduce capillary fragility, enhance lymphatic drainage, and promote wound healing in edema-related conditions such as venous ulcers and lymphedema.

Vitamin E: Vitamin E exerts antioxidant and anti-inflammatory effects, protecting against oxidative stress-induced tissue damage and inflammation in individuals with edema. Supplementation with vitamin E may help reduce edema-related inflammation, improve microcirculation, and enhance tissue perfusion, supporting overall vascular health and function.

Magnesium: Magnesium deficiency has been implicated in fluid retention, muscle cramps, and endothelial dysfunction, common features of edema-related conditions such as heart failure and venous insufficiency. Supplementation with magnesium can help restore electrolyte balance, promote vasodilation, and enhance lymphatic function, reducing edema severity and improving cardiovascular outcomes.

Omega-3 Fatty Acids: Omega-3 fatty acids, found in fatty fish, flaxseeds, chia seeds, and walnuts, exhibit anti-inflammatory and vasodilatory properties, beneficial for individuals with edema-related inflammation and microcirculatory dysfunction. Supplementation with omega-3 fatty acids may help reduce edema formation, improve lymphatic drainage, and support cardiovascular health, mitigating the risk of edema-related complications.

3. Herbal Remedies and Nutraceuticals:

Herbal remedies and nutraceuticals offer alternative therapeutic options for individuals with edema, harnessing the medicinal properties of botanical extracts, plant compounds, and dietary supplements to support lymphatic function, reduce inflammation, and enhance fluid balance regulation. These natural remedies provide adjunctive treatment options, promoting holistic approaches to edema management and overall well-being.

Horse Chestnut Extract: Horse chestnut extract, derived from the seeds of the Aesculus hippocastanum tree, exhibits venotonic and anti-inflammatory effects, beneficial for individuals with venous insufficiency, chronic venous edema, and varicose veins. Supplementation with horse chestnut extract may help improve venous tone, reduce capillary permeability, and alleviate symptoms of lower extremity edema.

Gotu Kola (Centella asiatica): Gotu kola, a traditional medicinal herb, has been used for centuries to promote wound healing, enhance collagen synthesis, and improve microcirculation. Gotu kola extracts contain active compounds, such as triterpenoids and asiaticoside, with anti-inflammatory, antioxidant, and venotonic properties, supporting lymphatic function and reducing edema severity in conditions such as lymphedema and venous insufficiency.

Bromelain: Bromelain, a proteolytic enzyme derived from pineapple stems, exhibits anti-inflammatory, fibrinolytic, and immune-modulating effects, beneficial for individuals with edema-related inflammation and tissue injury. Supplementation with bromelain may help reduce edema formation, alleviate pain and swelling, and promote tissue repair and regeneration in conditions such as post-surgical edema and sports injuries.

Rutin: Rutin, a flavonoid found in citrus fruits, buckwheat, and green tea, exerts antioxidant, anti-inflammatory, and venotonic effects, beneficial for individuals with venous insufficiency, capillary fragility, and chronic edema. Supplementation with rutin may help strengthen capillary walls, improve venous tone, and reduce edema severity, supporting overall vascular health and function.

Conclusion:

In conclusion, nutrition and nutraceuticals play a significant role in edema management, offering dietary strategies, micronutrient supplementation, and herbal remedies to support lymphatic function, reduce inflammation, and promote tissue healing. By adopting a balanced diet rich in essential nutrients, minimizing sodium intake, and incorporating specific nutraceuticals with anti-inflammatory and diuretic properties, individuals with edema can optimize fluid balance regulation, enhance vascular health, and improve overall well-being. Integrating nutrition-based approaches into comprehensive edema management plans complements conventional treatment modalities, promoting holistic approaches to optimize clinical outcomes and quality of life for individuals living with edema-related conditions.

Mind-Body Interventions: Yoga, Meditation, and Stress Reduction Techniques for Edema Management

Mind-body interventions, such as yoga, meditation, and stress reduction techniques, offer holistic approaches to edema management by addressing the interconnectedness of physical, mental, and emotional well-being. These practices promote relaxation, mindfulness, and self-awareness, empowering individuals with edema to cultivate resilience, reduce stress-related fluid retention, and enhance overall health. This exploration delves into the role of mind-body interventions in edema management, encompassing the physiological effects, therapeutic benefits, and practical applications of yoga, meditation, and stress reduction techniques, providing insights into integrative approaches to optimize fluid balance and support holistic healing.

1. Yoga for Edema Management:

Yoga, an ancient practice originating from India, integrates physical postures, breath control, and meditation to promote harmony between body, mind, and spirit. Yoga offers a gentle yet effective approach to edema management, combining stretching, strengthening, and relaxation techniques to improve circulation, lymphatic drainage, and stress resilience. Key components of yoga practice for edema management include:

Gentle Stretching: Yoga poses, such as forward bends, gentle twists, and inversions, promote venous return, lymphatic flow, and tissue mobilization, reducing fluid retention and promoting fluid redistribution away from the extremities.

Breath Awareness: Pranayama, or yogic breathing techniques, enhance oxygenation, relaxation, and parasympathetic nervous system activation, promoting vasodilation, diuresis, and stress reduction, essential for edema management and fluid balance regulation.

Mindfulness Meditation: Mindfulness meditation practices, integrated into yoga sessions, cultivate present-moment awareness, acceptance, and equanimity, reducing stress-related fluid retention, cortisol levels, and sympathetic nervous system activity, beneficial for individuals with edema-related stress and anxiety.

Yoga Nidra: Yoga nidra, or yogic sleep, induces deep relaxation, nervous system balance, and rejuvenation, promoting parasympathetic dominance, cellular repair, and tissue regeneration, essential for edema management and overall health.

Leg Elevation: Specific yoga poses, such as legs-up-the-wall pose (Viparita Karani), facilitate venous return, lymphatic drainage, and fluid mobilization from the lower extremities, reducing swelling and discomfort associated with edema.

2. Meditation for Edema Management:

Meditation, a mindfulness-based practice involving focused attention and awareness, offers therapeutic benefits for individuals with edema by reducing stress, enhancing relaxation, and promoting autonomic nervous system balance. Meditation cultivates a state of inner calm, emotional resilience, and mental clarity, facilitating self-regulation of physiological processes, including fluid balance regulation and lymphatic function. Key components of meditation practice for edema management include:

Focused Attention: Concentration meditation techniques, such as mindfulness of breath, body scan, or mantra repetition, enhance awareness, grounding, and present-moment focus, reducing stress-related sympathetic activation and fluid retention in individuals with edema.

Body Awareness: Body awareness meditation practices, such as mindful movement or progressive muscle relaxation, foster somatic awareness, tension release, and sensory integration, promoting lymphatic circulation, tissue decongestion, and fluid balance optimization.

Emotional Regulation: Loving-kindness meditation (Metta), compassion meditation (Karuna), and gratitude meditation (Anukampa) cultivate positive emotions, empathy, and resilience, reducing stress-related cortisol levels, inflammation, and fluid retention in individuals with edema-related emotional distress.

Visualization: Guided imagery and visualization techniques harness the power of the mind-body connection to promote healing, restoration, and cellular rejuvenation, facilitating lymphatic drainage, tissue repair, and fluid balance regulation in individuals with edema-related tissue damage or inflammation.

Breath Awareness: Breath-focused meditation practices, such as mindful breathing or diaphragmatic breathing, promote relaxation, parasympathetic activation, and respiratory efficiency, enhancing oxygenation, circulation, and lymphatic flow in individuals with edema-related respiratory compromise or venous insufficiency.

3. Stress Reduction Techniques for Edema Management:

Stress reduction techniques, including relaxation exercises, biofeedback, and cognitive-behavioral strategies, offer practical tools for managing stress-related fluid retention and promoting emotional well-being in individuals with edema. By cultivating relaxation, resilience, and coping skills, these techniques empower individuals to navigate life's challenges more effectively, mitigating the impact of stress on fluid balance regulation and lymphatic function. Key components of stress reduction techniques for edema management include:

Progressive Muscle Relaxation (PMR): PMR involves tensing and relaxing muscle groups systematically, promoting physical relaxation, stress reduction, and parasympathetic activation, essential for edema management and fluid balance regulation.

Deep Breathing Exercises: Deep breathing techniques, such as diaphragmatic breathing or paced breathing, induce relaxation, respiratory efficiency, and vagal tone, reducing sympathetic arousal, cortisol levels, and fluid retention in individuals with edema-related stress and anxiety.

Guided Imagery: Guided imagery scripts and recordings facilitate relaxation, visualization, and mental rehearsal, promoting positive emotions, immune modulation, and tissue healing in individuals with edema-related pain, inflammation, or tissue damage.

Mindfulness-Based Stress Reduction (MBSR): MBSR programs integrate mindfulness meditation, yoga, and cognitive-behavioral techniques to reduce stress, enhance resilience, and promote holistic well-being in individuals with chronic conditions, including edema-related disorders.

Cognitive Restructuring: Cognitive-behavioral strategies, such as cognitive restructuring or thought challenging, help individuals identify and modify maladaptive thoughts, beliefs, and behaviors contributing to stress-related fluid retention and emotional distress in edema management.

Conclusion:

In conclusion, mind-body interventions, including yoga, meditation, and stress reduction techniques, offer holistic approaches to edema management by addressing the interconnectedness of physical, mental, and emotional well-being. By promoting relaxation, mindfulness, and self-awareness, these practices empower individuals with edema to cultivate resilience, reduce stress-related fluid retention, and enhance overall health. Integrating mind-body interventions into comprehensive edema management plans complements conventional treatment modalities, fostering a holistic approach to optimize fluid balance, support lymphatic function, and promote holistic healing in individuals with edema-related conditions.

Traditional and Complementary Medicine Approaches for Edema Management

Traditional and complementary medicine approaches offer holistic and integrative strategies for managing edema, leveraging natural remedies, ancient healing practices, and cultural traditions to promote overall health and well-being. These approaches complement conventional medical treatments by addressing underlying imbalances, enhancing self-healing mechanisms, and optimizing physiological function. This exploration delves into the role of traditional and complementary medicine approaches in edema management, encompassing herbal medicine, acupuncture, Ayurveda, traditional Chinese medicine (TCM), and other indigenous healing modalities, providing insights into diverse cultural perspectives and integrative approaches to optimize fluid balance and support holistic healing.

1. Herbal Medicine:

Herbal medicine, also known as botanical medicine or phytotherapy, utilizes plant-based remedies to prevent and treat various health conditions, including edema. Herbal remedies offer natural alternatives to conventional medications, harnessing the therapeutic properties of medicinal plants to promote diuresis, reduce inflammation, and enhance lymphatic function. Key herbal remedies for edema management include:

Dandelion (Taraxacum officinale): Dandelion leaf and root have diuretic properties, promoting renal excretion of excess fluid and electrolytes, reducing edema severity, and supporting overall kidney function.

Horse Chestnut (Aesculus hippocastanum): Horse chestnut seed extract contains aescin, a compound with venotonic and anti-inflammatory effects, beneficial for individuals with venous insufficiency, chronic venous edema, and varicose veins.

Ginkgo Biloba: Ginkgo biloba extract improves microcirculation, reduces capillary permeability, and exhibits antioxidant properties, beneficial for individuals with edema-related inflammation, tissue damage, or cognitive impairment.

Bilberry (Vaccinium myrtillus): Bilberry fruit extract contains anthocyanins, flavonoids with antioxidant and anti-inflammatory effects, beneficial for individuals with venous insufficiency, capillary fragility, and chronic edema.

Bromelain: Bromelain, a proteolytic enzyme derived from pineapple stems, exhibits anti-inflammatory, fibrinolytic, and immune-modulating effects, beneficial for individuals with edema-related inflammation and tissue injury.

2. Acupuncture and Traditional Chinese Medicine (TCM):

Acupuncture and traditional Chinese medicine (TCM) offer holistic approaches to edema management by addressing underlying imbalances in the body's energy flow, or Qi, and promoting harmonization of organ systems. Acupuncture involves the insertion of thin needles into specific acupoints along meridians to stimulate Qi flow, regulate physiological functions, and promote homeostasis. Key TCM modalities for edema management include:

Acupuncture: Acupuncture points on the kidney, spleen, and liver meridians are targeted to regulate fluid metabolism, tonify Qi, and promote lymphatic drainage, reducing edema severity and enhancing overall vitality.

Herbal Formulas: TCM herbal formulas, such as Wu Ling San (Five-Ingredient Powder with Poria), Zhen Wu Tang (True Warrior Decoction), and Yi Yi Ren Tang (Coix Seed Decoction), address underlying imbalances in fluid metabolism, promoting diuresis, and reducing edema formation.

Dietary Therapy: TCM dietary principles emphasize the consumption of foods with cooling, draining, and harmonizing properties, such as leafy greens, cucumbers, melons, and mung beans, to support kidney function, promote urination, and reduce fluid retention.

Tuina Massage: Tuina, a TCM therapeutic massage technique, stimulates acupoints, meridians, and energy channels to promote Qi flow, lymphatic drainage, and tissue mobilization, reducing edema severity and promoting relaxation.

3. Ayurveda:

Ayurveda, an ancient system of medicine originating from India, offers personalized approaches to edema management based on individual constitutional types, or doshas, and imbalances in the body's elemental energies. Ayurvedic treatments aim to restore balance to the body, mind, and spirit by harmonizing the doshas and promoting optimal functioning of the bodily systems. Key Ayurvedic modalities for edema management include:

Panchakarma Therapy: Panchakarma, a detoxification and rejuvenation therapy, includes treatments such as Abhyanga (oil massage), Swedana (herbal steam therapy), and Virechana (therapeutic purgation), aimed at removing toxins, balancing doshas, and promoting lymphatic drainage.

Herbal Remedies: Ayurvedic herbal formulations, such as Triphala churna (Three-Fruit Powder), Punarnava (Boerhavia diffusa), and Guggulu (Commiphora mukul), promote diuresis, reduce inflammation, and support kidney function, beneficial for individuals with edema-related imbalances.

Dietary Recommendations: Ayurvedic dietary recommendations emphasize the consumption of foods with balancing properties for each dosha, such as warm, light, and dry foods for Kapha imbalance, to support digestion, metabolism, and elimination of excess fluids.

Yoga and Pranayama: Ayurvedic practices, such as yoga and pranayama (breath control techniques), promote circulation, lymphatic drainage, and balance of the doshas, reducing edema severity and enhancing overall vitality.

4. Indigenous Healing Modalities:

Indigenous healing modalities, rooted in cultural traditions and ancestral wisdom, offer holistic approaches to edema management by incorporating spiritual, ceremonial, and community-based practices to promote healing and wellness. Indigenous healing modalities honor the interconnectedness of all beings and the natural world, fostering harmony, reciprocity, and respect for the Earth. Key indigenous healing modalities for edema management include:

Medicinal Plants and Remedies: Indigenous cultures have deep knowledge of local plants and natural remedies used for centuries to promote health and treat various ailments, including edema. Traditional healers often employ plant-based medicines, herbal teas, and poultices to support lymphatic function, reduce inflammation, and promote healing.

Ceremonial Healing Practices: Ceremonial healing practices, such as sweat lodges, smudging ceremonies, and plant medicine ceremonies, offer opportunities for spiritual purification, emotional release, and energetic alignment, essential for healing on the physical, mental, and emotional levels.

Community Support and Connection: Indigenous healing traditions emphasize the importance of community support, reciprocity, and connection in promoting healing and wellness. Healing circles, support groups, and communal gatherings provide opportunities for individuals with edema to share experiences, receive guidance, and cultivate a sense of belonging and solidarity.

Mindfulness and Connection to Nature: Indigenous healing modalities emphasize mindfulness, presence, and connection to the natural world as essential aspects of health and healing. Practices such as nature walks, meditation in natural settings, and rituals honoring the elements foster a deep sense of connection, grounding, and reverence for the Earth, supporting overall well-being and vitality.

Conclusion:

In conclusion, traditional and complementary medicine approaches offer diverse and culturally rich strategies for edema management, integrating natural remedies, ancient healing practices, and indigenous wisdom to promote holistic health and well-being. Herbal medicine, acupuncture, Ayurveda, traditional Chinese medicine (TCM), and indigenous healing modalities provide holistic and integrative approaches to optimize fluid balance, support lymphatic function, and promote holistic healing in individuals with edema-related conditions. By embracing the principles of holistic healing and honoring the interconnectedness of body, mind, and spirit, traditional and complementary medicine approaches empower individuals to reclaim their health, vitality, and resilience on the path to wellness.

Printed in Great Britain
by Amazon